SJOGREN'S SYNDROME DIET COOKBOOK

FOR BEGINNERS

Ease Your Symptoms with Nourishing, Anti-Inflammatory Recipes and Practical Tips for a Healthier Lifestyle

Kingsley Klopp

To show our appreciation for your purchase, we're delighted to offer you these special bonuses as a heartfelt thank you.

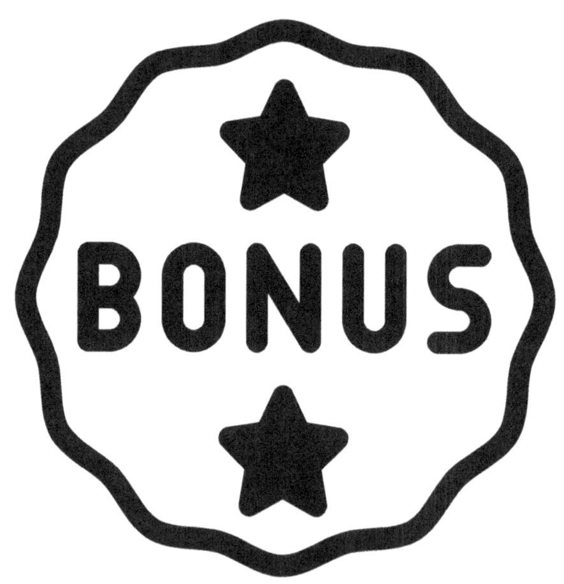

1. A Food Tracker Journal
2. Downloadable E-BOOK featuring full-color images of finished recipes

Table of Contents

Soup & Stew Recipes

Smoothies

Dear cherished reader,

We extend a hearty welcome to you as you set out on this healthy journey with the "**Sjogren's Syndrome Diet Cookbook**," and we share your excitement about finding dishes that will not only satisfy your palate but also provide solace and respite from the symptoms of Sjogren's Syndrome.

However, as we venture together into the world of culinary healing, it's crucial to acknowledge the beautifully unique tapestry that is our health and nutritional needs. Just as each of us has our own stories and struggles, so too do our bodies respond differently to various foods and dietary adjustments. With this in mind, we gently remind you that the recipes within these pages are starting points on your journey to wellness. They are your canvas, awaiting personal touches, substitutions, and adjustments to align perfectly with your body's specific requirements and preferences.

We wholeheartedly encourage you to embrace the art of customization. Feel empowered to tweak ingredients, swap out elements that may not suit you, and experiment with flavors that bring you joy and comfort, all while keeping your nutritional needs in the spotlight. Your body's response is the ultimate guide; listen to it with care and attention. In addition, we recognize the importance of professional guidance on this journey. If ever you find yourself at a crossroads, unsure of how a certain dietary change might affect your Sjogren's Syndrome or overall health, we urge you to consult with your healthcare provider. Their expertise can offer invaluable insights and ensure that your dietary choices contribute positively to your health management plan.

Please also bear in mind that the nutritional information provided alongside each recipe is approximate. Factors such as the specific brands of ingredients used, their freshness, and even the way individual ingredients are processed can affect the final nutritional content of each dish. We've done our best to provide accurate estimates, but consider these numbers a guide rather than an exact science.

Furthermore, if this cookbook has enhanced your cooking and dining experience, we would love to read about your journey in an Amazon review. Conversely, if you encounter any issues with the recipes, please feel free to reach out to us at **kloppkingsley@gmail.com.** We are dedicated to assisting you throughout your culinary adventure.

Introduction

Welcome to the **Sjogren's Syndrome Diet Cookbook for Beginner**s, your compassionate guide through the transformative journey of managing and living with Sjogren's Syndrome through the power of nutrition. Whether you're newly diagnosed, a longtime warrior against the condition, or caring for someone who is, you've taken an essential step towards embracing a lifestyle that can significantly ease your symptoms and enhance your overall well-being.

Living with Sjogren's Syndrome, a complex autoimmune disorder that predominantly attacks the body's moisture-producing glands, presents a unique set of challenges. From the persistent dryness of the eyes and mouth to potential complications involving other organs, the impact of Sjogren's extends far beyond mere discomfort —it can profoundly affect one's quality of life. However, amidst these challenges lies an empowering truth: the food you eat can play a pivotal role in managing your symptoms and reclaiming your health. The idea that *"food is medicine"* holds particular resonance for those navigating the complexities of autoimmune conditions. Our aim with this cookbook is not just to provide you with recipes but to offer a new lens through which to view your diet and its profound impact on your symptoms and overall health. This is a journey of discovery, where each meal brings you closer to understanding how the right foods can moisturize from the inside out, reduce inflammation, and energize your body and spirit.

You will discover more than just a compilation of recipes as you read through these pages. You'll uncover the foundations of a diet designed to combat the dryness and discomfort that come with Sjogren's. We've carefully selected dishes that are not only hydrating and easy to consume but also rich in nutrients that are known to support immune system regulation and reduce inflammation. From smooth, soothing soups to hydrating smoothies and nutrient-packed main dishes, each recipe is a stepping stone towards a more comfortable and enjoyable daily life.

This book, however, serves as a companion in addition to a cookbook. It's here to guide you through the uncertainties that come with adjusting your diet, offering practical advice on meal planning, grocery shopping, and making the most of each ingredient. We understand that change isn't always easy, especially when it comes to food, which is so deeply intertwined with culture, comfort, and tradition. That's why we've approached each recipe with flexibility in mind, offering substitutions and variations to accommodate different tastes, dietary restrictions, and the ever-changing availability of ingredients.

So, let's begin this journey together. Open your mind (and your kitchen) to the possibilities that lie ahead. With each recipe, you'll learn not just how to cook, but how to nourish your body and soothe your symptoms, turning mealtime into a healing ritual. Let's turn the page and start cooking our way to better health.

PART 1

THE BASICS OF SJOGREN'S SYNDROME

Sjogren's Syndrome is an autoimmune disease characterized primarily by its effects on the body's moisture-producing glands. This condition often leads to significant dryness, particularly affecting the eyes and mouth, but it can also impact other parts of the body, including the skin, joints, lungs, kidneys, and nervous system. It is essential for everyone who has been diagnosed with Sjogren's Syndrome to understand the illness, including their family, caregivers, and the medical professionals who assist them.

What is Sjogren's Syndrome?
Sjogren's Syndrome is a long-term autoimmune disorder where the immune system mistakenly attacks parts of the body, particularly the glands that produce tears and saliva. This results in the primary symptoms: dry eyes (keratoconjunctivitis sicca) and dry mouth (xerostomia). While these are the most common manifestations, Sjogren's can be systemic, affecting various organs and causing a wide range of symptoms.

Causes and Risk Factors
The exact cause of Sjogren's Syndrome is unknown, but a combination of genetic, environmental, and possibly hormonal factors is believed to contribute to its development. Viral infections have also been studied as potential triggers. The condition is more commonly diagnosed in women than men and typically occurs in people over the age of 40, although it can develop at any age.

Treatment and Management
While there is no cure for Sjogren's Syndrome, the condition can be managed through a combination of lifestyle adjustments and medical treatments aimed at alleviating symptoms and preventing complications. Treatment strategies may include:
- Artificial tears and saliva substitutes to relieve dryness
- Medications to stimulate saliva production

- Immunosuppressive drugs in severe cases
- Good oral hygiene to prevent dental complications
- Regular eye exams and dental visits

Lifestyle and Dietary Considerations
Patients with Sjogren's Syndrome can also benefit from dietary changes and lifestyle adjustments to manage symptoms. Staying hydrated, avoiding dry environments, using humidifiers, and following a balanced diet rich in omega-3 fatty acids and anti-inflammatory foods can support overall health and reduce symptom severity.

Sjogren's Syndrome is a complex condition that requires a comprehensive management strategy encompassing medical treatment, lifestyle adjustments, and support. With proper management, people with Sjogren's can lead active, fulfilling lives. Awareness and understanding are key to navigating the challenges posed by the condition, emphasizing the importance of education, support networks, and ongoing research into effective treatments.

Symptoms and Diagnosis

Symptoms of Sjogren's Syndrome

Sjogren's Syndrome primarily affects the body's moisture-producing glands, leading to the hallmark symptoms of dry eyes and dry mouth. However, it can also cause a range of other symptoms due to its systemic nature, impacting various parts of the body. Here's a closer look at the symptoms:

- **Dry Eyes (Keratoconjunctivitis Sicca):** Individuals may experience a gritty or burning sensation in the eyes, sensitivity to light, blurred vision, or eye fatigue. This occurs because the condition affects the glands that produce tears, leading to decreased tear production and increased tear evaporation.
- **Dry Mouth (Xerostomia):** This can feel like a sticky, dry sensation in the mouth, leading to difficulties in swallowing, speaking, and tasting. It can also increase the risk of dental decay, gingivitis (gum inflammation), and mouth infections, such as thrush.
- **Dry Skin:** Many people with Sjogren's Syndrome also experience dryness of the skin, which can lead to itching and rashes.
- **Joint Pain, Swelling, and Stiffness:** Similar to other autoimmune disorders, Sjogren's can cause rheumatoid symptoms, affecting the joints.
- **Dryness in Other Areas:** This can include vaginal dryness, dry cough, and dryness in the nasal passages, which can lead to nosebleeds.
- **Fatigue and Brain Fog:** Chronic fatigue and difficulty concentrating, often referred to as "brain fog," are common, affecting the quality of life.
- **Other Systemic Symptoms:** Less commonly, Sjogren's can affect the kidneys, lungs, liver, pancreas, and nervous system, leading to a wide array of symptoms from organ dysfunction.

Diagnosis of Sjogren's Syndrome

Diagnosing Sjogren's Syndrome can be complex and usually involves multiple steps, as symptoms often overlap with those of other conditions, including other autoimmune disorders.

- **Medical History and Physical Examination**: A healthcare provider will review the patient's medical history and symptoms and perform a physical exam, focusing on the eyes and mouth.
- **Blood Tests**: Certain blood tests can detect the presence of antibodies commonly found in people with Sjogren's Syndrome, such as anti-Ro (SSA) and anti-La (SSB) antibodies. Blood tests can also reveal markers of inflammation and indicators of organ function to assess the impact of the syndrome on other parts of the body.
- **Schirmer's Test**: This simple test measures tear production by placing a small strip of filter paper under the lower eyelid. Reduced tear production is a sign of dry eye syndrome associated with Sjogren's.
- **Salivary Gland Function Tests**: These tests can measure how much saliva the mouth produces and may include sialography, which involves taking an X-ray of the salivary ducts after injecting a dye.
- **Lip Biopsy**: A small sample of tissue from the salivary glands in the lip may be taken and examined under a microscope for signs of inflammation consistent with Sjogren's Syndrome.
- **Ocular Surface Staining**: Special eye drops with dyes are used to identify areas of damage on the surface of the eye, which can be indicative of dry eye syndrome.

Due to the overlap of symptoms with other conditions and the variability of symptoms among individuals, diagnosing Sjogren's Syndrome can be challenging. It often requires a combination of tests and a high index of suspicion. Early diagnosis and treatment are crucial to managing symptoms effectively and reducing the risk of complications. Treatment typically focuses on relieving symptoms and may include medications to increase moisture production, manage pain and inflammation, and address specific organ involvement.

How Diet Can Help

Diet plays a crucial role in managing Sjogren's Syndrome, a chronic autoimmune condition characterized by dryness, particularly of the eyes and mouth, and potentially affecting other parts of the body. While there's no specific diet that can cure Sjogren's, certain dietary approaches can help alleviate symptoms, improve overall health, and reduce inflammation associated with the condition. Here's how diet can help in managing Sjogren's Syndrome:

1. Hydration

- **Maximizing Intake:** Staying well-hydrated is essential for managing dryness. Drinking plenty of water throughout the day helps alleviate dry mouth and supports overall bodily functions.
- **Hydrating Foods:** Incorporating fruits and vegetables with high water content, such as cucumbers, celery, watermelon, and oranges, can also contribute to hydration.

2. Anti-inflammatory Foods

- **Omega-3 Fatty Acids:** Foods rich in omega-3 fatty acids, like salmon, flaxseeds, and walnuts, have anti-inflammatory properties that can help reduce systemic inflammation and potentially improve symptoms.
- **Antioxidant-rich Foods:** Fruits and vegetables, whole grains, nuts, and seeds are packed with antioxidants that combat inflammation. Berries, spinach, and sweet potatoes are particularly beneficial.

3. Avoiding Inflammatory Foods

- **Processed and Sugary Foods:** Reducing the intake of processed foods, sugars, and trans fats, which can promote inflammation, might help manage symptoms better.
- **Gluten and Dairy:** Some individuals with autoimmune disorders find that gluten and dairy exacerbate their symptoms. Though evidence is anecdotal, experimenting with reducing or eliminating these foods may be beneficial for some.

4. Sialogogues (Saliva Stimulating Foods)

- **Sour and Tart Foods:** Consuming foods that naturally stimulate saliva production, such as lime, and other citrus fruits (in moderatio to avoid dental erosion), can help manage dry mouth
- **Chewing Gums and Lozenges:** Sugar-free chewing gum or lozenges can stimulate saliva flow. Look for products containing xylitol, which can also help reduce the risk of tooth decay.

5. Supplements

- **Vitamin D:** Autoimmune disease sufferers, including those with Sjogren's Syndrome, often have lower levels of vitamin D. Supplementing with vitamin D, under a doctor's supervision, can support immune function and bone health.
- **Omega-3 Supplements:** For those who don't consume enough omega-3s through their diet, fish oil supplements can be an alternative source.

6. Gut Health

- **Probiotics and Prebiotics:** Maintaining a healthy gut microbiome is important for overall health and immunity. Probiotics (found in yogurt, kefir, and sauerkraut) and prebiotics (found in foods like garlic, onions, and bananas) support gut health, which can influence inflammation and immune response.

7. Dietary Adjustments for Specific Symptoms

- **Soft and Moist Foods:** For those with severe dry mouth, eating moist, soft foods can make chewing and swallowing more comfortable. Adding broths, sauces, or gravies can help.
- **Avoiding Irritants:** Spicy, acidic, or very salty foods can irritate dry mouths and should be consumed in moderation or avoided.

While diet alone cannot cure Sjogren's Syndrome, it plays a significant role in managing symptoms and improving quality of life. A balanced, nutrient-rich diet that emphasizes hydration, anti-inflammatory foods, and dietary adjustments to ease specific symptoms can support overall health and may reduce the severity of Sjogren's symptoms. It's also important for individuals with Sjogren's Syndrome to work with healthcare providers, including nutritionists, to tailor dietary strategies to their specific needs, ensuring they receive adequate nutrition while managing their symptoms.

PART 2
NUTRITIONAL GUIDELINES FOR SJOGREN'S SYNDROME

Essential Nutrients and Vitamins

For people with Sjogren's Syndrome, an autoimmune disorder characterized by dryness of the eyes, mouth, and other glands, maintaining a diet rich in specific nutrients and vitamins is crucial. These essential nutrients and vitamins can help mitigate symptoms, reduce inflammation associated with the autoimmune response, and support overall health. An overview of the main vitamins and nutrients that are good for people with Sjogren's syndrome is provided below:

1. **Omega-3 Fatty Acids**
   - **Benefits:** Omega-3 fatty acids are known for their anti-inflammatory properties, which can help reduce the systemic inflammation seen in autoimmune disorders like Sjogren's Syndrome.
   - **Sources:** Fatty fish (such as salmon, mackerel, and sardines), flaxseeds, chia seeds, and walnuts are excellent sources of omega-3 fatty acids.
2. **Vitamin D**
   - **Benefits:** Vitamin D plays a critical role in immune system regulation and bone health. Some studies suggest that higher levels of vitamin D are associated with a reduced risk of autoimmune diseases.
   - **Sources:** Few foods naturally contain vitamin D; fatty fish, fish liver oils, and fortified foods are among the best sources. Sunlight exposure is also a significant source of vitamin D.

3. Antioxidants

- **Vitamin C**: This vitamin supports the immune system and has antioxidant properties, it also help in the production of saliva.
    - **Sources**: Citrus fruits, strawberries, bell peppers, and kiwis are rich in vitamin C.
- **Vitamin E**: Vitamin E is an antioxidant that protects body tissue from damage and supports immune health.
    - **Sources**: Almonds, hazelnuts, sunflower seeds, and green leafy vegetables are good sources of vitamin E.
- **Selenium**: This mineral has antioxidant properties that help protect cells from damage.
    - **Sources**: Brazil nuts, seafood, and meats contain selenium.

4. B Vitamins

- **Benefits**: B vitamins, including B6, B12, and folate, play a role in nerve function and could help with the neurological symptoms sometimes associated with Sjogren's Syndrome.
- **Sources**: Whole grains, legumes, bananas, potatoes, and lean meats are sources of B vitamins.

5. Zinc

- **Benefits**: Zinc contributes to immune function, wound healing, and tissue repair, which can be beneficial for managing Sjogren's symptoms.
- **Sources**: Meat, shellfish, legumes, seeds, and nuts are excellent sources of zinc.

6. Fluids

- **Benefits**: Adequate hydration is crucial for managing the dryness associated with Sjogren's. Water helps maintain moisture levels in the body and can alleviate symptoms of dry mouth and eyes.
- **Sources**: Apart from drinking water, consuming foods with high water content like fruits and vegetables can contribute to hydration.

7. Probiotics and Prebiotics

- **Benefits**: These support gut health, which is essential for immune function. A healthy gut microbiota may influence overall inflammation and immune response.
- **Sources**: Probiotics are found in fermented foods like yogurt, kefir, and sauerkraut. Prebiotics are in foods like garlic, onions, and asparagus.

8. Fiber

- **Benefits:** Fiber supports digestive health and can help prevent the constipation that might be exacerbated by certain Sjogren's medications.
- **Sources:** Whole grains, vegetables, fruits, and legumes are rich in fiber.

Implementing Nutritional Strategies

Incorporating these nutrients into a balanced diet can help manage symptoms of Sjogren's Syndrome and support overall health. However, it's essential to remember that individual nutritional needs can vary. Consulting with healthcare professionals, such as a dietitian or nutritionist, who understands Sjogren's Syndrome, can provide tailored advice and dietary plans to meet personal health needs and preferences.

Moreover, while dietary adjustments can play a significant role in symptom management, they should complement, not replace, the treatment plan prescribed by healthcare providers.

Foods to Include and Avoid

Foods to Include

1. Hydration-Boosting Foods

- **Water:** The most crucial element for hydration. Drinking plenty of water throughout the day helps mitigate dryness symptoms.
- **Cucumbers, Celery, and Watermelon:** These and other fruits and vegetables with high water content can aid in keeping the body hydrated.

2. Omega-3 Fatty Acids

- **Fatty Fish:** Salmon, mackerel, and sardines are rich in omega-3s, which can help reduce inflammation.
- **Flaxseeds and Chia Seeds:** Plant-based sources of omega-3s, beneficial for those who do not consume fish.

3. Antioxidant-Rich Foods

- **Berries, Cherries, and Plums:** Packed with antioxidants, these fruits can help combat oxidative stress and inflammation.
- **Green Leafy Vegetables:** Spinach, kale, and Swiss chard are excellent sources of vitamins A, C, E, and K.

4. Whole Grains

- **Quinoa, Brown Rice, and Oats:** These provide fiber, which can help maintain a healthy digestive system, reducing the risk of constipation, which can be a concern due to decreased fluid intake.

5. Anti-Inflammatory Spices and Herbs

- **Turmeric and Ginger:** Known for their anti-inflammatory properties, they can be added to meals to help reduce systemic inflammation.

6. Moist and Soft Foods

- **Stews, Soups, and Smoothies:** Easy to consume for individuals experiencing severe dryness and can be packed with nutrients if prepared with the right ingredients.

Foods to Avoid

1. Dehydrating Foods and Drinks
- **Caffeinated Beverages:** Coffee, tea, and some sodas can exacerbate dryness by increasing urine output.
- **Alcoholic Beverages:** Alcohol is a diuretic and can lead to further dehydration.

2. High-Sodium Foods
- **Processed Foods:** Often high in sodium, which can promote dehydration, these should be limited or avoided.
- **Salty Snacks:** Chips, crackers, and pretzels can aggravate dry mouth.

3. Acidic Foods and Beverages
- **Citrus Fruits and Juices:** While beneficial in moderation for their vitamin C content, they can irritate dry mouth and should be consumed carefully.
- **Tomatoes and Tomato-based Products:** Can also irritate a dry mouth due to their acidity.

4. Spicy Foods
- **Hot Peppers and Spicy Dishes:** These can exacerbate mouth discomfort and dryness.

5. Sugary Foods and Beverages
- **Sweets and Sugary Drinks:** Can contribute to dental problems, especially important to avoid given the increased risk of dental decay with dry mouth.

6. Dry and Crunchy Foods
- **Crackers, Dry Breads, and Chips:** Can be difficult to consume for those with dry mouth and can pose a risk for choking or discomfort.

BREAKFAST RECIPES

1. Moist Banana Pancakes

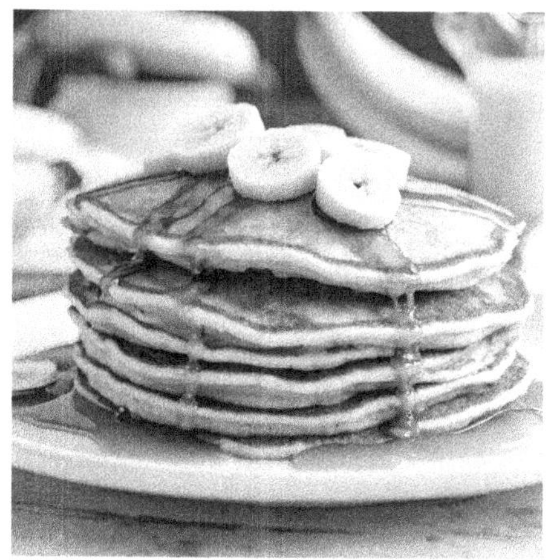

Ingredients:

- 2 ripe bananas
- 1 cup all-purpose flour
- 1 tablespoon sugar
- 1 teaspoon baking powder
- 1/2 teaspoon baking soda
- 1/4 teaspoon salt
- 1 egg, beaten
- 1 cup buttermilk
- 2 tablespoons unsalted butter, melted
- 1 teaspoon vanilla extract

Instructions:

1. In a large bowl, mash the ripe bananas with a fork until smooth.
2. Add the beaten egg, buttermilk, melted butter, and vanilla extract to the bananas. Stir until well combined.
3. In a separate bowl, whisk together the flour, sugar, baking powder, baking soda, and salt.
4. Gradually mix the dry ingredients into the wet ingredients until just combined; be careful not to overmix.
5. Heat a non-stick pan over medium heat and lightly grease it with butter or oil.
6. Pour 1/4 cup of batter for each pancake onto the hot pan. Cook until bubbles form on the surface, then flip and cook until golden brown.
7. Serve warm.

Nutrition Info per Serving (serves 4):

- Calories: 290
- Protein: 7g
- Carbohydrates: 45g
- Fat: 9g
- Sodium: 410mg
- Fiber: 3g

Cooking Time: 20 minutes

2. Vegetable Soup
Ingredients:
- 2 tablespoons olive oil
- 1 onion, diced
- 2 carrots, peeled and diced
- 2 stalks celery, diced
- 2 cloves garlic, minced
- 1 zucchini, diced
- 1 potato, peeled and diced
- 4 cups vegetable broth
- 1 can (14 oz) diced tomatoes
- 1 teaspoon dried oregano
- 1 teaspoon dried basil
- Salt and pepper to taste
- 1 cup chopped spinach or kale

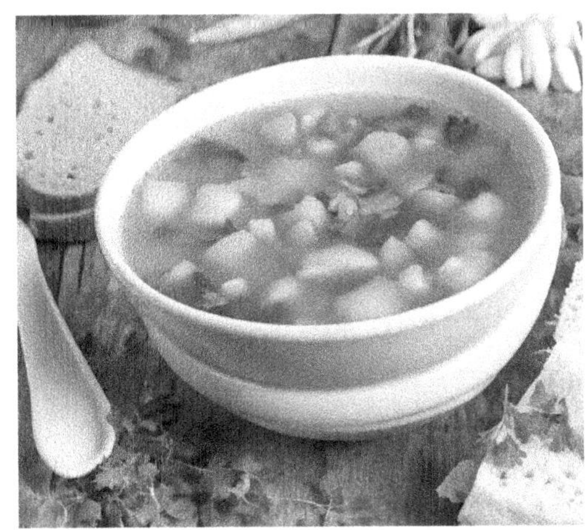

Instructions:
1. In a large pot, heat the olive oil over medium heat. Add the onion, carrots, and celery, and cook until they start to soften, about 5 minutes.
2. Add the garlic, zucchini, and potato, and cook for another 2 minutes.
3. Pour in the vegetable broth and diced tomatoes. Bring to a boil, then reduce heat and simmer for 20 minutes.
4. Add the oregano, basil, salt, and pepper. Stir in the spinach or kale, and cook until the greens are wilted, about 2 minutes.
5. Serve hot.

Nutrition Info per Serving (serves 6):
- Calories: 120
- Protein: 3g
- Carbohydrates: 18g
- Fat: 4g
- Sodium: 650mg
- Fiber: 4g

Cooking Time: 30 minutes

3. Applesauce

Ingredients:

- 4 apples, peeled, cored, and chopped
- 3/4 cup water
- 1/4 cup sugar (adjust to taste)
- 1/2 teaspoon ground cinnamon

Instructions:

1. In a saucepan, combine the apples, water, sugar, and cinnamon. Bring to a boil, then reduce heat.
2. Cover and simmer for 15-20 minutes or until apples are soft.
3. Use a potato masher or blender to puree the mixture to your desired consistency.
4. Serve warm or chilled.

Nutrition Info per Serving (serves 4):

- Calories: 110
- Protein: 0g
- Carbohydrates: 29g
- Fat: 0g
- Sodium: 2mg
- Fiber: 5g

Cooking Time: 25 minutes

4. Peaches and Cream Oatmeal

Ingredients:

- 1 cup rolled oats
- 2 cups water or milk for creamier texture
- 1 pinch salt
- 1 cup sliced peaches (fresh or canned in juice)
- 1/2 cup heavy cream or coconut cream
- 2 tablespoons honey or maple syrup
- 1/2 teaspoon vanilla extract

Instructions:

1. Bring water or milk to a boil in a medium saucepan. Add oats and salt, reducing heat to a simmer.
2. Cook for 5 minutes, stirring occasionally, until oats are soft.
3. Stir in sliced peaches, heavy or coconut cream, honey or maple syrup, and vanilla extract.
4. Serve warm.

Nutrition Info per Serving (serves 2):

- Calories: 420
- Protein: 10g
- Carbohydrates: 63g
- Fat: 15g
- Sodium: 80mg
- Fiber: 6g

Cooking Time: 10 minutes

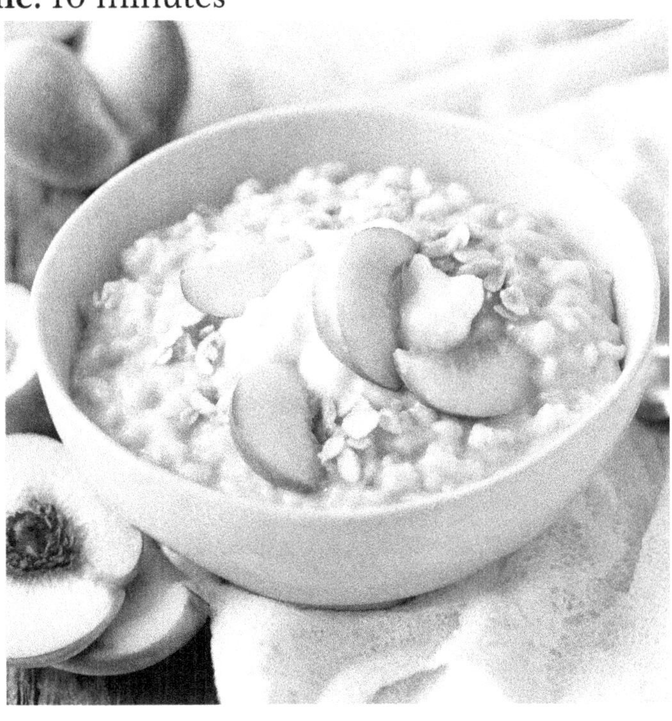

5. Tofu Scramble

Ingredients:

- 1 block (14 oz) firm tofu, drained and crumbled
- 2 tablespoons olive oil
- 1/2 onion, diced
- 1 bell pepper, diced
- 1 teaspoon turmeric
- 1/2 teaspoon garlic powder
- Salt and pepper to taste
- 1/4 cup nutritional yeast (optional for a cheesy flavor)
- 1 tablespoon soy sauce or tamari

Instructions:

1. Heat olive oil in a skillet over medium heat. Add onion and bell pepper, sautéing until soft.
2. Add crumbled tofu, turmeric, garlic powder, salt, and pepper. Cook for 5-7 minutes, stirring frequently.
3. Stir in nutritional yeast and soy sauce. Cook for another 2-3 minutes.
4. Serve warm, optionally with toasted bread.

Nutrition Info per Serving (serves 3):

- Calories: 230
- Protein: 16g
- Carbohydrates: 9g
- Fat: 15g
- Sodium: 300mg
- Fiber: 3g

Cooking Time: 15 minutes

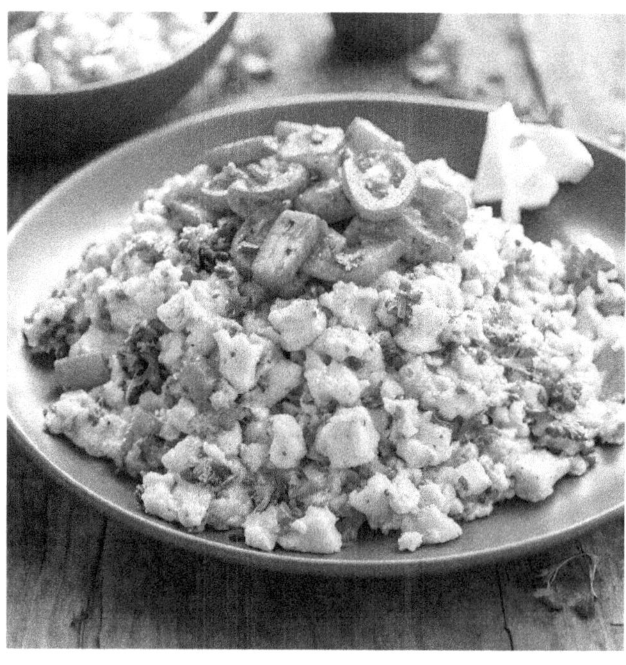

6. Porridge

Ingredients:
- 1 cup steel-cut oats
- 4 cups water or milk for creaminess
- 1/4 teaspoon salt
- Toppings: sliced banana, berries, honey, cinnamon

Instructions:
1. In a large saucepan, bring water or milk to a boil. Add oats and salt, reducing heat to a simmer.
2. Cook uncovered, stirring occasionally, for 25-30 minutes until oats are tender.
3. Serve with your choice of toppings.

Nutrition Info per Serving (serves 4):
- Calories: 150 (without toppings)
- Protein: 6g
- Carbohydrates: 27g
- Fat: 2.5g
- Sodium: 150mg
- Fiber: 4g

Cooking Time: 30 minutes

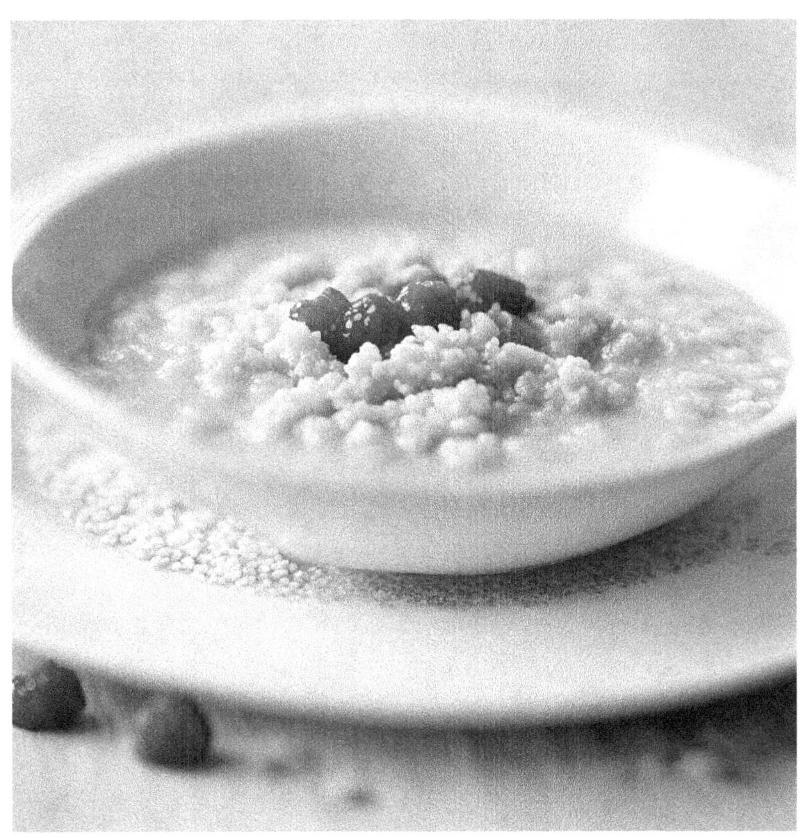

7. Soft French Toast

Ingredients:

- 4 slices of soft bread (brioche or challah works well)
- 2 eggs
- 1/2 cup milk
- 1 teaspoon vanilla extract
- 1/2 teaspoon cinnamon
- Butter for frying
- Maple syrup for serving

Instructions:

1. In a shallow dish, whisk together eggs, milk, vanilla extract, and cinnamon.
2. Heat a skillet over medium heat and melt a bit of butter.
3. Dip each bread slice in the egg mixture, ensuring both sides are coated.
4. Fry each side until golden brown, about 2-3 minutes per side.
5. Serve warm with maple syrup.

Nutrition Info per Serving (serves 2):

- Calories: 320
- Protein: 12g
- Carbohydrates: 45g
- Fat: 10g
- Sodium: 430mg
- Fiber: 2g

Cooking Time: 15 minutes

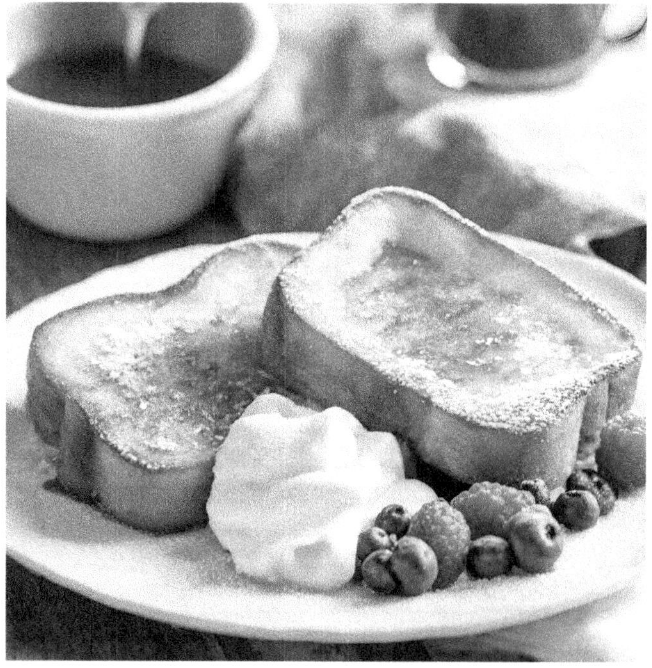

8. Warm Berry Compote

Ingredients:

- 2 cups mixed berries (fresh or frozen)
- 1/4 cup orange juice
- 2 tablespoons honey or maple syrup
- 1 teaspoon vanilla extract
- 1/2 teaspoon ground cinnamon

Instructions:

1. In a saucepan, combine berries, orange juice, honey or maple syrup, vanilla extract, and cinnamon.
2. Cook over medium heat for 10-15 minutes, stirring occasionally, until the berries are soft and the sauce has thickened slightly.
3. Serve warm over oatmeal, pancakes, or yogurt.

Nutrition Info per Serving (serves 4):

- Calories: 70
- Protein: 1g
- Carbohydrates: 18g
- Fat: 0g
- Sodium: 5mg
- Fiber: 3g

Cooking Time: 15 minutes

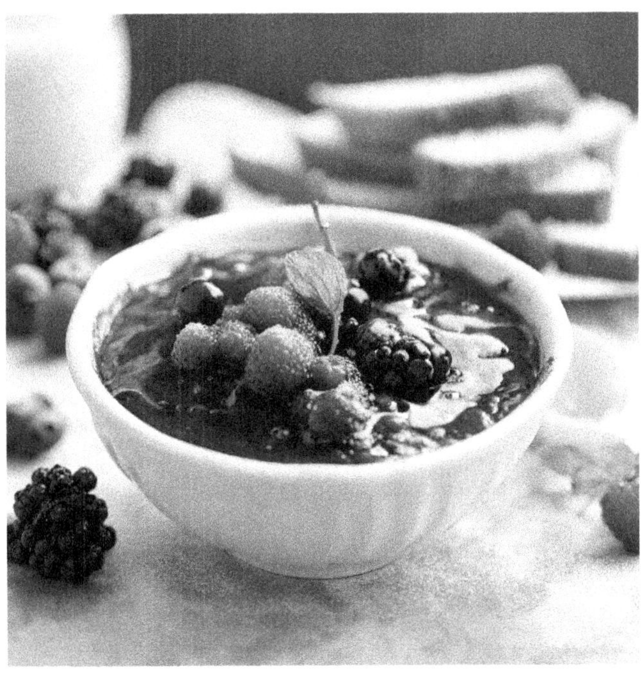

9. Egg Muffins

Ingredients:

- 6 eggs
- 1/4 cup milk
- Salt and pepper to taste
- 1/2 cup shredded cheese (optional)
- 1/2 cup diced vegetables (spinach, bell peppers, onions)
- Cooking spray or oil for greasing

Instructions:

1. Preheat your oven to 350°F (175°C). Grease a muffin tin with cooking spray or oil.
2. In a bowl, whisk together eggs, milk, salt, and pepper.
3. Stir in cheese and diced vegetables.
4. Pour the egg mixture into the muffin tin, filling each cup about 3/4 full.
5. Bake for 20-25 minutes, or until the muffins are set and lightly golden on top.
6. Let cool for a few minutes before serving.

Nutrition Info per Serving (serves 6):

- Calories: 100 (with cheese)
- Protein: 9g
- Carbohydrates: 2g
- Fat: 7g
- Sodium: 200mg
- Fiber: 0.5g

Cooking Time: 30 minutes

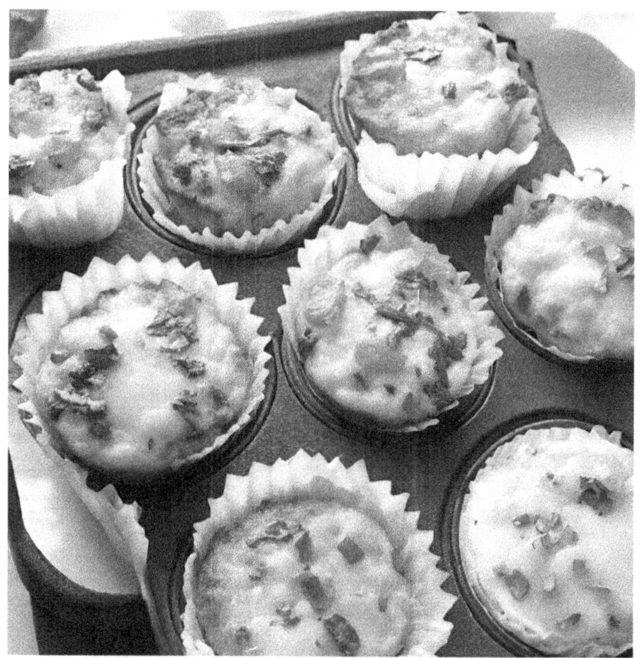

10. Zucchini Muffins

Ingredients:

- 1 1/2 cups all-purpose flour
- 3/4 cup sugar
- 1 teaspoon baking soda
- 1 teaspoon ground cinnamon
- 1/2 teaspoon salt
- 1 egg, beaten
- 1/2 cup vegetable oil
- 1/4 cup milk
- 1 tablespoon lemon juice
- 1 teaspoon vanilla extract
- 1 cup grated zucchini
- 1/2 cup chopped nuts or raisins (optional)

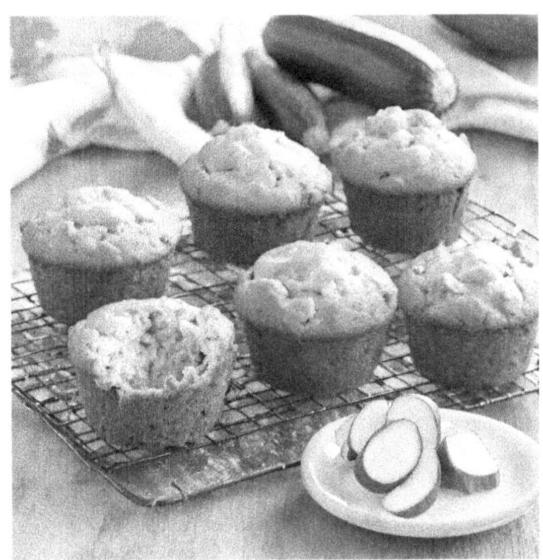

Instructions:

1. Preheat oven to 350°F (175°C). Grease or line a muffin tin.
2. In a large bowl, combine flour, sugar, baking soda, cinnamon, and salt.
3. In another bowl, mix together egg, oil, milk, lemon juice, and vanilla extract.
4. Stir the wet ingredients into the dry ingredients just until moistened. Fold in grated zucchini and nuts or raisins if using.
5. Fill muffin cups 3/4 full with batter.
6. Bake for 20-25 minutes, or until a toothpick inserted into the center comes out clean.
7. Let cool in pan for 10 minutes, then transfer to a wire rack to cool completely.

Nutrition Info per Serving (serves 12):

- Calories: 200 (with nuts)
- Protein: 3g
- Carbohydrates: 27g
- Fat: 9g
- Sodium: 220mg
- Fiber: 1g

Cooking Time: 35 minutes

11. Banana Bread

Ingredients:

- 3 ripe bananas, mashed
- 1/3 cup melted butter
- 3/4 cup sugar
- 1 egg, beaten
- 1 teaspoon vanilla extract
- 1 teaspoon baking soda
- Pinch of salt
- 1 1/2 cups of all-purpose flour

Instructions:

1. Preheat oven to 350°F (175°C). Grease a 4x8-inch loaf pan.
2. In a mixing bowl, stir together mashed bananas and melted butter.
3. Mix in sugar, egg, and vanilla.
4. Sprinkle baking soda and salt over the mixture and mix in.
5. Add flour last, mix just until incorporated. Pour mixture into prepared loaf pan.
6. Bake for 50 to 60 minutes, or until a toothpick inserted into the center comes out clean.
7. Let bread cool in the pan for a few minutes, then turn out onto a wire rack to cool completely.

Nutrition Info per Serving (serves 10):

- Calories: 220
- Protein: 3g
- Carbohydrates: 37g
- Fat: 7g
- Sodium: 230mg
- Fiber: 1g

Cooking Time: 1 hour 10 minutes

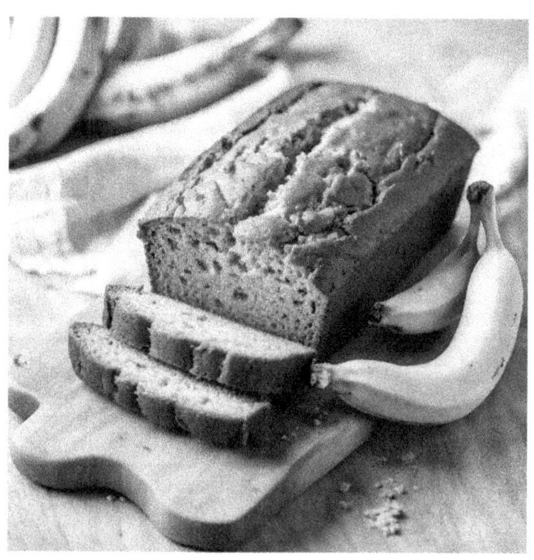

12. Steamed Vegetables

Ingredients:

- 1 cup broccoli florets
- 1 cup carrot slices
- 1 cup zucchini slices
- Salt and pepper to taste
- 1 tablespoon olive oil
- 1 teaspoon lemon juice

Instructions:

1. Fill a pot with a few inches of water and bring to a boil. Place a steamer basket above the water.
2. Add the broccoli, carrots, and zucchini to the basket. Cover and steam for 5-7 minutes, or until vegetables are tender but still slightly crisp.
3. Transfer the vegetables to a bowl. Toss with olive oil, lemon juice, salt, and pepper.
4. Serve warm.

Nutrition Info per Serving (serves 4):

- Calories: 60
- Protein: 2g
- Carbohydrates: 8g
- Fat: 3.5g
- Sodium: 75mg
- Fiber: 3g

Cooking Time: 12 minutes

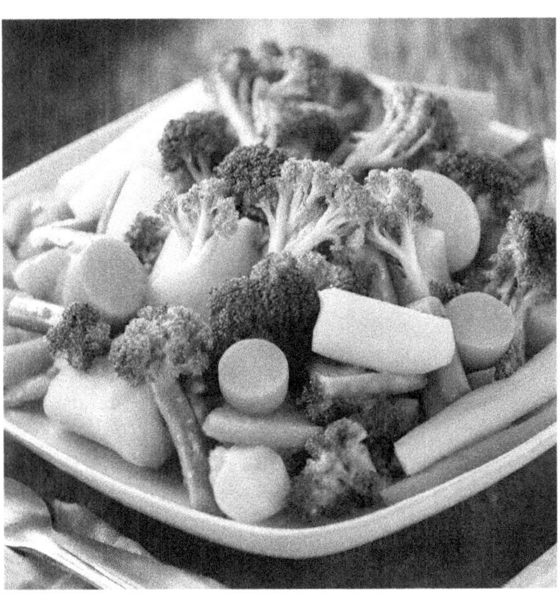

13. Pumpkin Smoothie

Ingredients:

- 1 cup pumpkin puree (canned or fresh)
- 1 banana
- 1 cup almond milk (or milk of choice)
- 1/2 teaspoon pumpkin pie spice
- 1 tablespoon maple syrup
- Ice cubes

Instructions:

1. Combine all ingredients in a blender.
2. Blend on high until smooth and creamy.
3. Serve immediately, garnished with a sprinkle of pumpkin pie spice if desired.

Nutrition Info per Serving (serves 2):

- Calories: 150
- Protein: 2g
- Carbohydrates: 35g
- Fat: 1g
- Sodium: 80mg
- Fiber: 5g

Cooking Time: 5 minutes

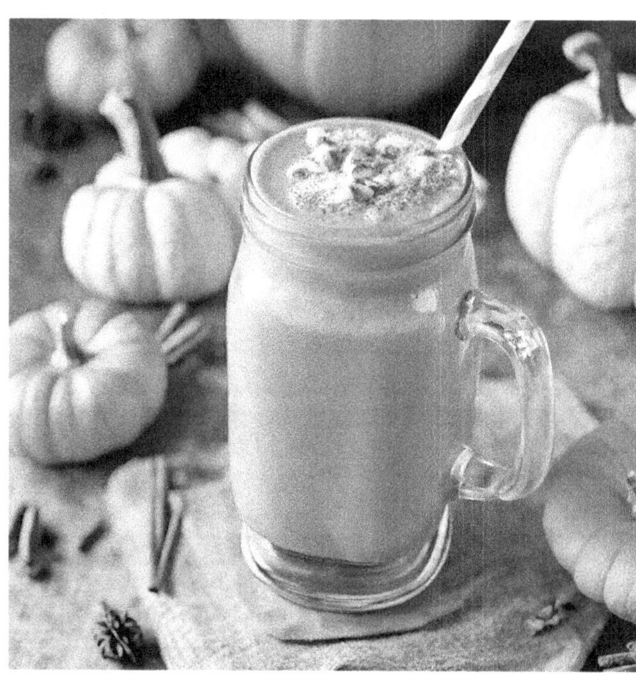

14. Creamy Polenta

Ingredients:

- 1 cup polenta (cornmeal)
- 4 cups water or broth for more flavor
- 1/2 teaspoon salt
- 1/4 cup grated Parmesan cheese
- 2 tablespoons butter

Instructions:

1. Bring water or broth to a boil in a large saucepan. Gradually whisk in polenta and salt.
2. Reduce heat to low and cook, stirring frequently, until polenta is thick and creamy, about 15-20 minutes.
3. Remove from heat and stir in Parmesan cheese and butter until well combined.
4. Serve warm.

Nutrition Info per Serving (serves 4):

- Calories: 250
- Protein: 6g
- Carbohydrates: 38g
- Fat: 8g
- Sodium: 450mg
- Fiber: 2g

Cooking Time: 25 minutes

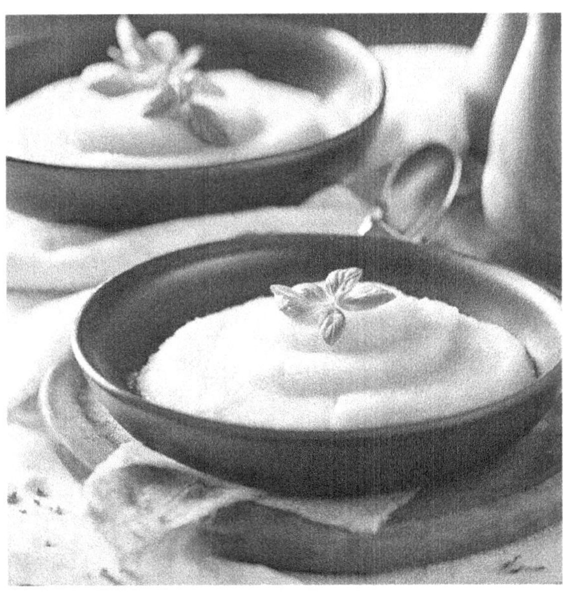

15. Mashed Avocado

Ingredients:
- 2 ripe avocados
- Juice of 1 lime
- Salt and pepper to taste

Instructions:
1. Cut the avocados in half, remove the pits, and scoop the flesh into a bowl.
2. Add lime juice, salt, and pepper.
3. Mash with a fork to your desired consistency.
4. Serve immediately, perfect as a spread on soft toast or as a side.

Nutrition Info per Serving (serves 4):
- Calories: 160
- Protein: 2g
- Carbohydrates: 9g
- Fat: 14g
- Sodium: 10mg
- Fiber: 7g

Cooking Time: 5 minutes

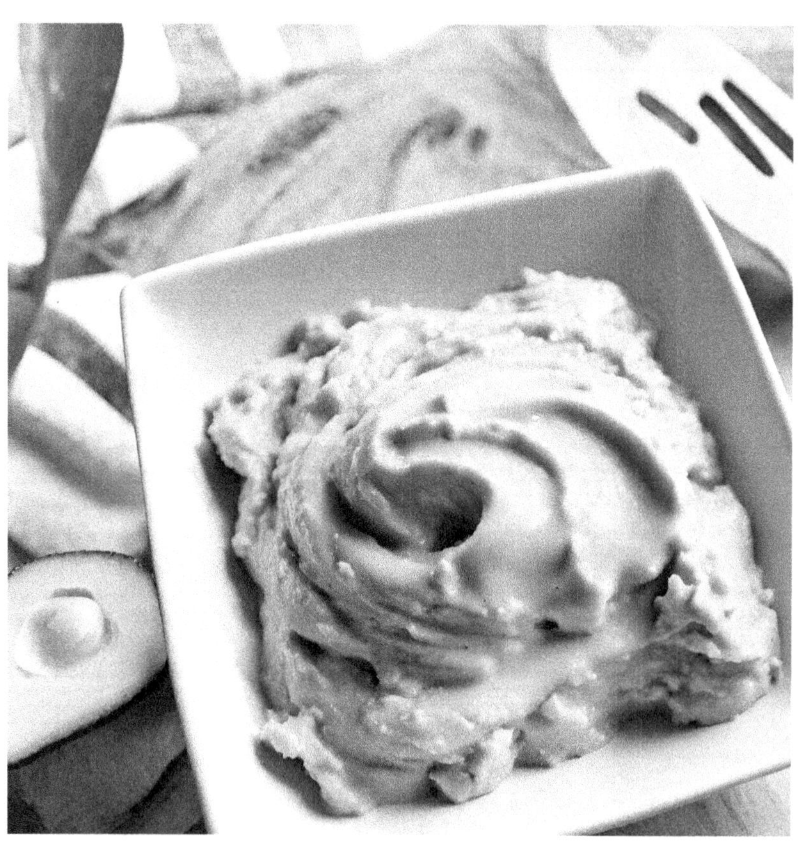

17. Homemade Ricotta Cheese

Ingredients:

- 4 cups whole milk
- 1 cup heavy cream
- 1/2 teaspoon salt
- 3 tablespoons lemon juice

Instructions:

1. Combine milk, cream, and salt in a large saucepan. Slowly bring the mixture to a full, but gentle, boil over medium heat, stirring occasionally.
2. Add lemon juice, then reduce heat to low and simmer, stirring gently, until the mixture curdles, about 2 minutes.
3. Pour the mixture into a colander lined with a few layers of cheesecloth set over a large bowl. Let drain for 1 hour.
4. After draining, the ricotta can be transferred to a container. It will keep in the refrigerator for up to 4 days.
5. Serve as part of a breakfast dish, on toast, or with fruit.

Nutrition Info per Serving (serves 6):

- Calories: 180
- Protein: 8g
- Carbohydrates: 6g
- Fat: 14g
- Sodium: 200mg
- Fiber: 0g

Cooking Time: 1 hour 15 minutes (including draining time)

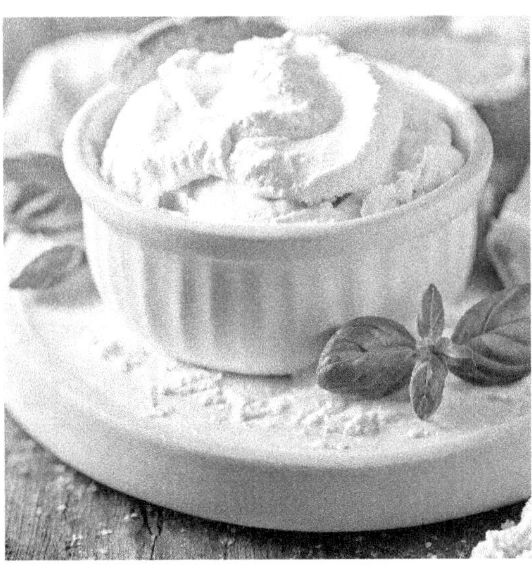

18. Cottage Cheese

Ingredients:

- 1 gallon low-fat milk
- 3/4 cup white vinegar or lemon juice
- 1 teaspoon salt

Instructions:

1. Pour the milk into a large pot, and slowly heat it on the stove over medium heat until it reaches 120°F (49°C), stirring occasionally.
2. Add the vinegar or lemon juice and stir gently for 2 minutes. The milk will separate into curds and whey.
3. Remove the pot from heat and let it sit undisturbed for 30 minutes.
4. Line a colander with cheesecloth and place it over a large bowl. Pour the mixture into the colander to separate the curds from the whey.
5. Once drained, transfer the curds to a bowl. Add salt and break the curds up with a spoon or your fingers until you reach the desired consistency.
6. Store in the refrigerator in an airtight container for up to 1 week.
7. Serve as part of your breakfast, with fruit or on toast.

Nutrition Info per Serving (serves 8):

- Calories: 150
- Protein: 28g
- Carbohydrates: 12g
- Fat: 2g
- Sodium: 400mg
- Fiber: 0g

Cooking Time: 1 hour (including resting and draining time)

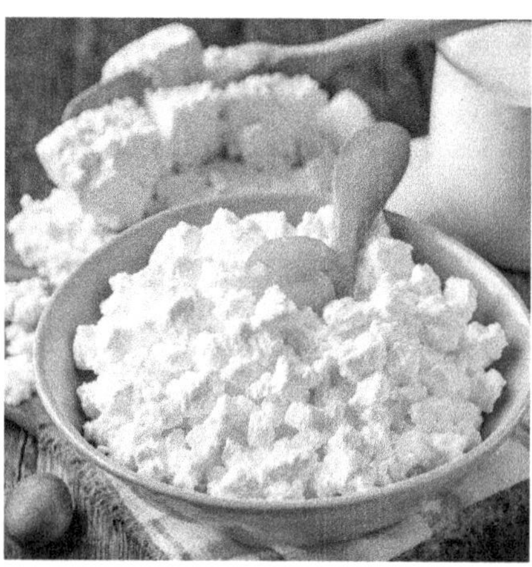

19. Greek Yogurt Parfait

Ingredients:
- 2 cups Greek yogurt
- 1/2 cup granola
- 1 cup mixed berries (such as strawberries, blueberries, and raspberries)
- 2 tablespoons honey or maple syrup
- 1/4 teaspoon vanilla extract (optional)

Instructions:
1. In a bowl, mix the Greek yogurt with vanilla extract and a tablespoon of honey or maple syrup for added sweetness, if desired.
2. In serving glasses or bowls, layer the Greek yogurt, granola, and mixed berries.
3. Drizzle the remaining honey or maple syrup over the top.
4. Serve immediately or refrigerate until ready to eat.

Nutrition Info per Serving (serves 4):
- Calories: 220
- Protein: 15g
- Carbohydrates: 30g
- Fat: 5g
- Sodium: 50mg
- Fiber: 2g

Cooking Time: 10 minutes

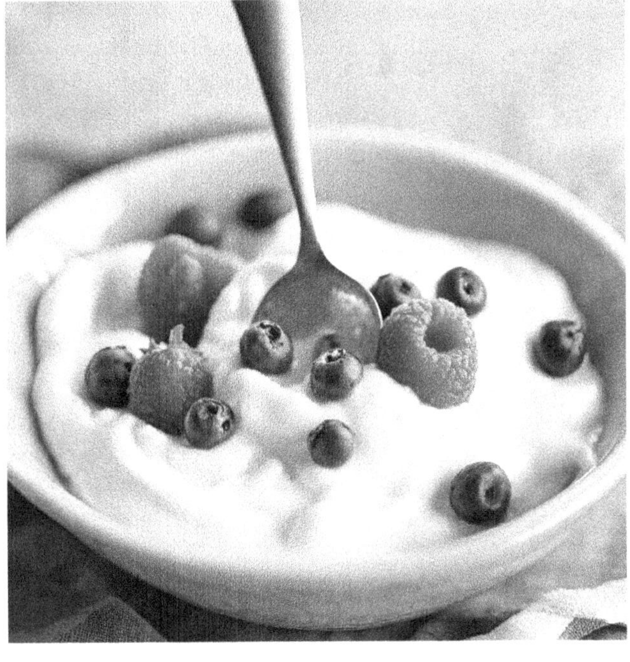

20. Quinoa Porridge

Ingredients:

- 1 cup quinoa, rinsed
- 2 cups almond milk or milk of choice
- 1/2 teaspoon cinnamon
- 1 apple, peeled and diced
- 2 tablespoons maple syrup or honey
- 1/4 cup raisins or dried cranberries
- Nuts or seeds for topping (optional)

Instructions:

1. Combine quinoa, almond milk, and cinnamon in a medium saucepan. Bring to a boil.
2. Reduce heat to low, cover, and simmer for 15 minutes.
3. Add the diced apple and raisins. Cook for another 5 minutes, or until quinoa is soft and most of the liquid is absorbed.
4. Stir in maple syrup or honey.
5. Serve hot, garnished with nuts or seeds if desired.

Nutrition Info per Serving (serves 4):

- Calories: 270
- Protein: 6g
- Carbohydrates: 55g
- Fat: 3g
- Sodium: 80mg
- Fiber: 5g

Cooking Time: 25 minutes

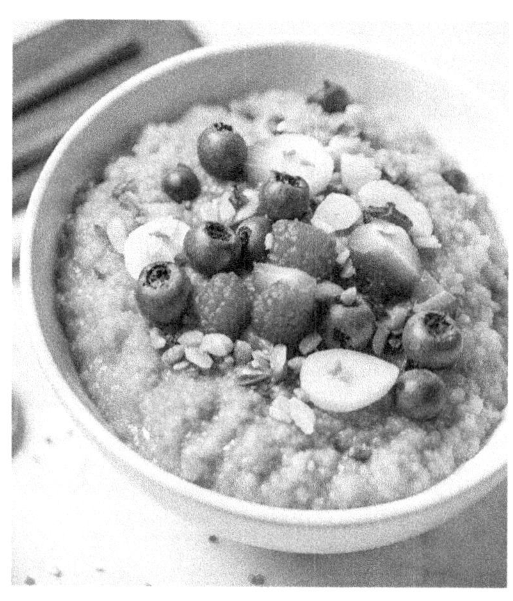

21. Smoothie Bowls

Ingredients:
- 2 cups frozen mixed berries
- 1 banana, sliced and frozen
- 1/2 cup Greek yogurt
- 1/2 cup almond milk or liquid of choice
- Toppings: sliced fruit, granola, coconut flakes, nuts, seeds, honey or maple syrup

Instructions:
1. In a blender, combine frozen berries, frozen banana, Greek yogurt, and almond milk. Blend until smooth.
2. Pour the smoothie into bowls.
3. Top with your choice of sliced fruit, granola, coconut flakes, nuts, and seeds. Drizzle with honey or maple syrup.
4. Serve immediately.

Nutrition Info per Serving (serves 2):
- Calories: 350
- Protein: 10g
- Carbohydrates: 60g
- Fat: 8g
- Sodium: 70mg
- Fiber: 8g

Cooking Time: 10 minutes

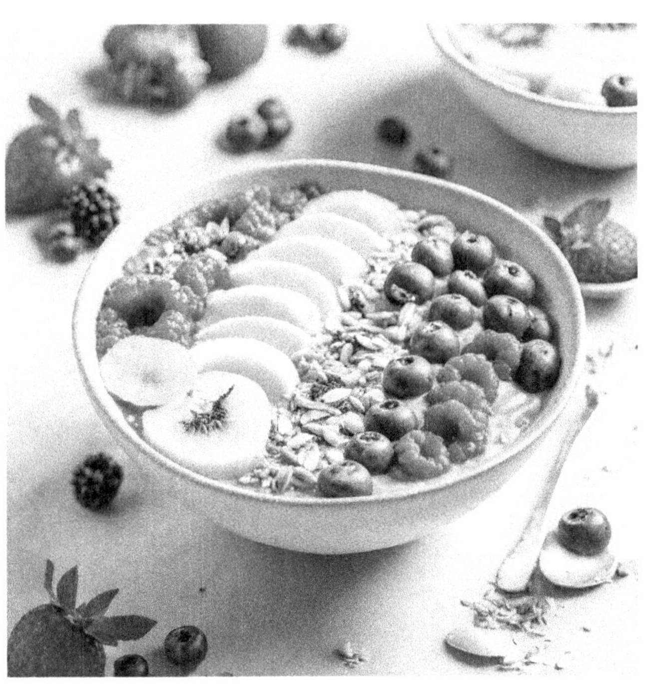

22. Overnight Oats

Ingredients:

- 1 cup rolled oats
- 1 cup almond milk or milk of choice
- 1/2 cup Greek yogurt
- 2 tablespoons chia seeds
- 2 tablespoons maple syrup or honey
- 1/2 teaspoon vanilla extract
- Toppings: fresh fruit, nuts, seeds, nut butter

Instructions:

1. In a bowl or jar, combine rolled oats, almond milk, Greek yogurt, chia seeds, maple syrup or honey, and vanilla extract. Stir well.
2. Cover and refrigerate overnight, or for at least 6 hours.
3. Before serving, stir the oats and add a little more milk if too thick. Add your favorite toppings.
4. Serve cold or at room temperature.

Nutrition Info per Serving (serves 2):

- Calories: 350
- Protein: 12g
- Carbohydrates: 55g
- Fat: 10g
- Sodium: 80mg
- Fiber: 8g

Cooking Time: Overnight (plus 5 minutes prep time)

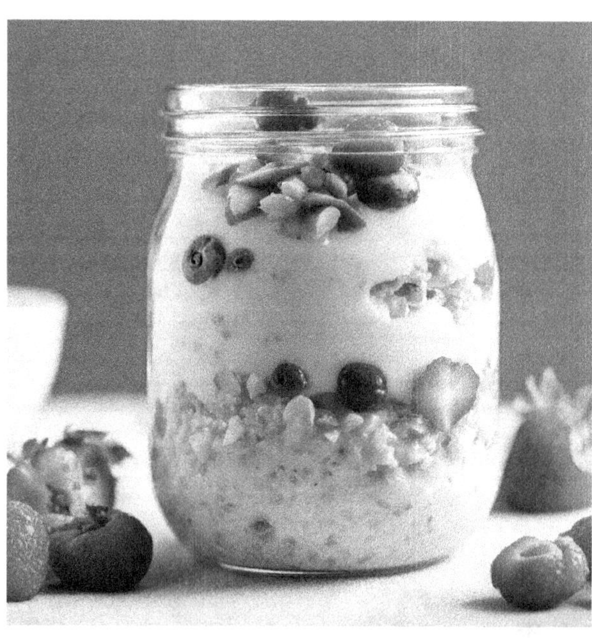

VEGETABLES

1. Cucumber Ribbon Salad

Ingredients:

- 2 large cucumbers
- 1/4 cup rice vinegar
- 2 tablespoons olive oil
- 1 tablespoon honey or maple syrup
- Salt and pepper to taste
- 1/4 cup thinly sliced red onion
- 2 tablespoons chopped fresh dill

Instructions:

1. Use a vegetable peeler or mandoline to slice the cucumbers into long, thin ribbons.
2. In a large bowl, whisk together rice vinegar, olive oil, honey, salt, and pepper.
3. Add cucumber ribbons and red onion to the dressing. Toss gently to combine.
4. Chill in the refrigerator for at least 30 minutes before serving. Just before serving, sprinkle with fresh dill.

Nutrition Info per Serving (serves 4):

- Calories: 110
- Protein: 1g
- Carbohydrates: 10g
- Fat: 7g
- Sodium: 10mg
- Fiber: 1g

Cooking Time: 40 minutes (including chilling time)

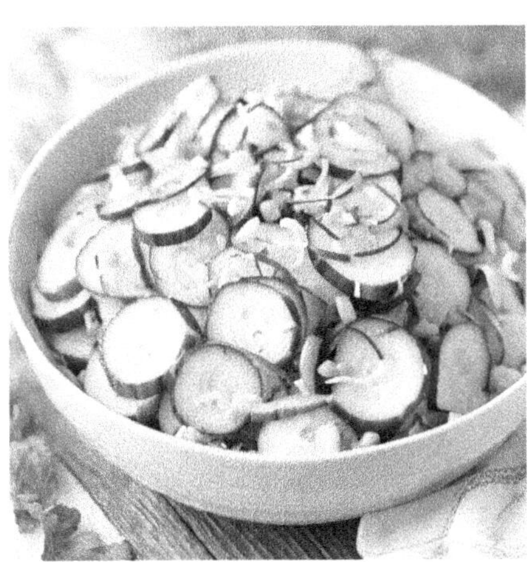

2. Shredded Carrot and Beet Salad

Ingredients:

- 2 medium carrots, peeled
- 2 medium beets, peeled
- 2 tablespoons olive oil
- 1 tablespoon lemon juice
- 1 teaspoon honey or maple syrup
- Salt and pepper to taste
- 1/4 cup chopped walnuts (optional)
- 2 tablespoons chopped fresh parsley

Instructions:

1. Use a grater or food processor to shred the carrots and beets.
2. In a large bowl, whisk together olive oil, lemon juice, honey, salt, and pepper.
3. Add shredded carrots and beets to the bowl and toss to coat with the dressing.
4. Chill in the refrigerator for at least 30 minutes to allow flavors to meld.
5. Before serving, sprinkle with walnuts (if using) and fresh parsley.

Nutrition Info per Serving (serves 4):

- Calories: 140
- Protein: 2g
- Carbohydrates: 14g
- Fat: 9g
- Sodium: 70mg
- Fiber: 3g

Cooking Time: 40 minutes (including chilling time)

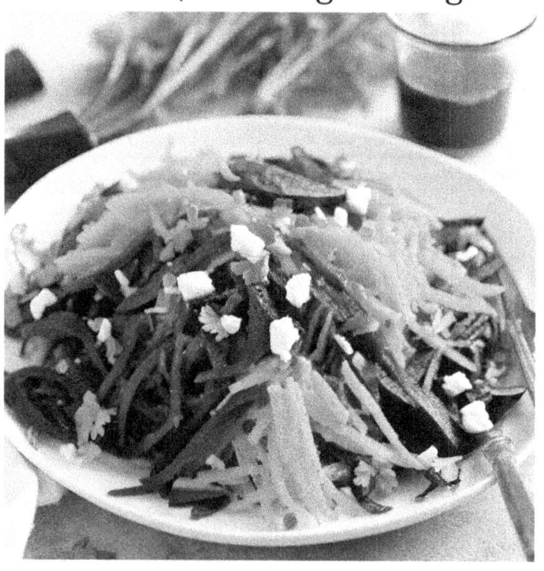

3. Zucchini Noodle Caprese

Ingredients:

- 2 large zucchinis
- 1 cup cherry tomatoes, halved
- 8 ounces fresh mozzarella cheese, cut into small cubes
- 1/4 cup fresh basil leaves, torn
- 2 tablespoons olive oil
- 1 tablespoon balsamic vinegar
- Salt and pepper to taste

Instructions:

1. Use a spiralizer or a vegetable peeler to create zucchini noodles (zoodles).
2. In a large bowl, combine zoodles, cherry tomatoes, mozzarella, and basil.
3. Drizzle with olive oil and balsamic vinegar. Season with salt and pepper.
4. Toss gently to combine.
5. Serve immediately or chill in the refrigerator for up to 30 minutes before serving.

Nutrition Info per Serving (serves 4):

- Calories: 250
- Protein: 14g
- Carbohydrates: 8g
- Fat: 19g
- Sodium: 270mg
- Fiber: 2g

Cooking Time: 15 minutes

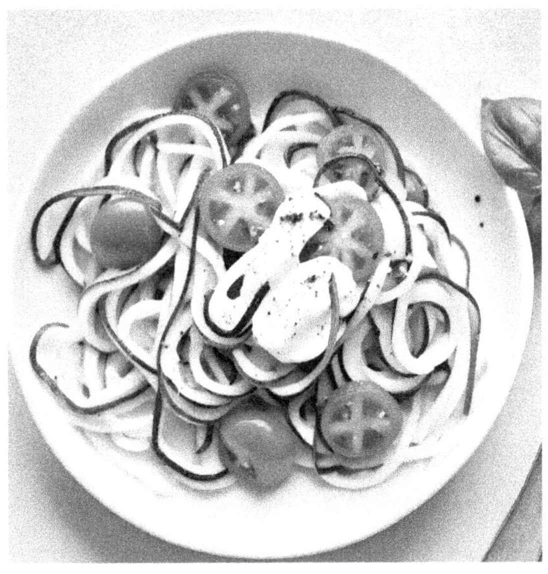

4. Watermelon and Feta Salad

Ingredients:

- 4 cups cubed watermelon
- 1 cup crumbled feta cheese
- 1/2 cup sliced red onion
- 1/4 cup chopped fresh mint
- 2 tablespoons olive oil
- 1 tablespoon lime juice
- Salt and pepper to taste

Instructions:

1. In a large bowl, combine watermelon, feta cheese, red onion, and fresh mint.
2. Drizzle with olive oil and lime juice. Season with salt and pepper.
3. Toss gently to combine.
4. Serve immediately or chill in the refrigerator for up to an hour before serving.

Nutrition Info per Serving (serves 4):

- Calories: 180
- Protein: 5g
- Carbohydrates: 15g
- Fat: 12g
- Sodium: 320mg
- Fiber: 1g

Cooking Time: 15 minutes

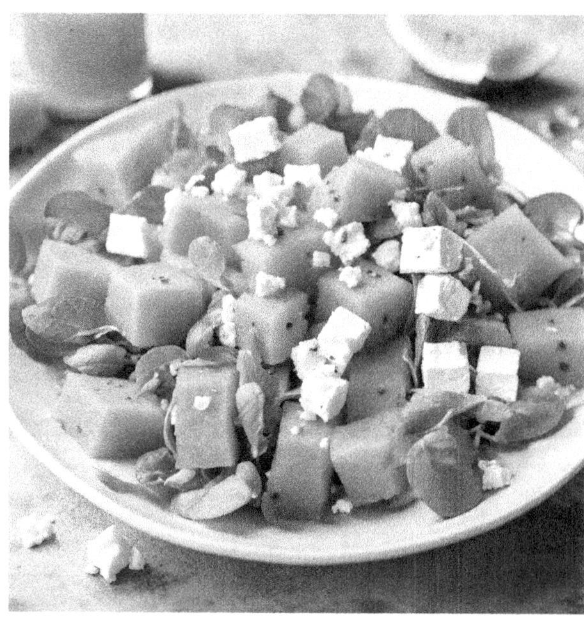

5. Creamy Butternut Squash Soup

Ingredients:

- 1 large butternut squash (about 2 pounds), peeled, seeded, and cubed
- 1 tablespoon olive oil
- 1 medium onion, chopped
- 3 cloves garlic, minced
- 4 cups vegetable broth
- 1 teaspoon salt
- 1/2 teaspoon black pepper
- 1/2 cup coconut milk

Instructions:

1. In a large pot, heat olive oil over medium heat. Add onion and garlic, and sauté until soft, about 5 minutes.
2. Add cubed butternut squash, vegetable broth, salt, and pepper. Bring to a boil, then reduce heat and simmer until squash is tender, about 20 minutes.
3. Use an immersion blender to purée the soup until smooth. Stir in coconut milk and heat through.
4. Serve hot.

Nutrition Info per Serving (serves 6):

- Calories: 150
- Protein: 2g
- Carbohydrates: 25g
- Fat: 5g
- Sodium: 800mg
- Fiber: 4g

Cooking Time: 35 minutes

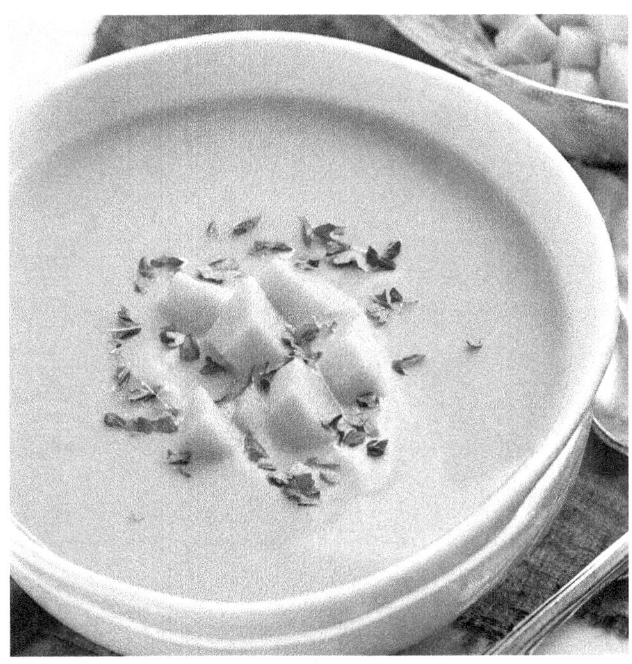

6. Carrot Ginger Soup

Ingredients:

- 1 tablespoon olive oil
- 1 onion, chopped
- 2 tablespoons grated fresh ginger
- 2 pounds carrots, peeled and chopped
- 4 cups vegetable broth
- Salt and pepper to taste
- 1 cup coconut milk

Instructions:

1. In a large pot, heat olive oil over medium heat. Add onion and ginger, and cook until onion is translucent, about 5 minutes.
2. Add carrots, vegetable broth, salt, and pepper. Bring to a boil, then reduce heat and simmer until carrots are tender, about 30 minutes.
3. Purée the soup using an immersion blender or in batches in a blender until smooth.
4. Stir in coconut milk and heat through before serving.

Nutrition Info per Serving (serves 6):

- Calories: 180
- Protein: 2g
- Carbohydrates: 27g
- Fat: 7g
- Sodium: 700mg
- Fiber: 6g

Cooking Time: 45 minutes

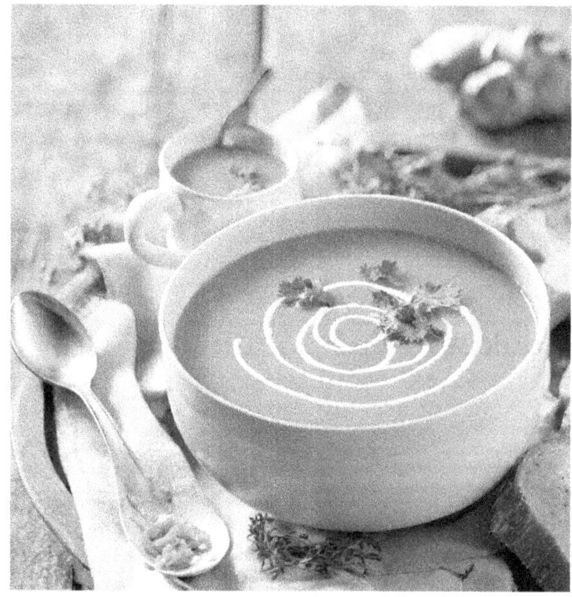

7. Zucchini Basil Soup

Ingredients:

- 2 tablespoons olive oil
- 1 onion, chopped
- 2 cloves garlic, minced
- 4 cups chopped zucchini
- 4 cups vegetable broth
- 1/2 cup fresh basil leaves, plus more for garnish
- Salt and pepper to taste
- 1/2 cup heavy cream or coconut cream

Instructions:

1. In a large pot, heat olive oil over medium heat. Add onion and garlic, and cook until softened.
2. Add zucchini and vegetable broth, bringing to a boil. Lower heat and simmer until zucchini is tender, about 15 minutes.
3. Add basil, salt, and pepper. Purée the soup using an immersion blender or in a regular blender until smooth.
4. Return soup to the pot, stir in cream or coconut cream, and heat through.
5. Garnish with fresh basil leaves before serving.

Nutrition Info per Serving (serves 6):

- Calories: 140
- Protein: 2g
- Carbohydrates: 8g
- Fat: 11g
- Sodium: 650mg
- Fiber: 2g

Cooking Time: 30 minutes

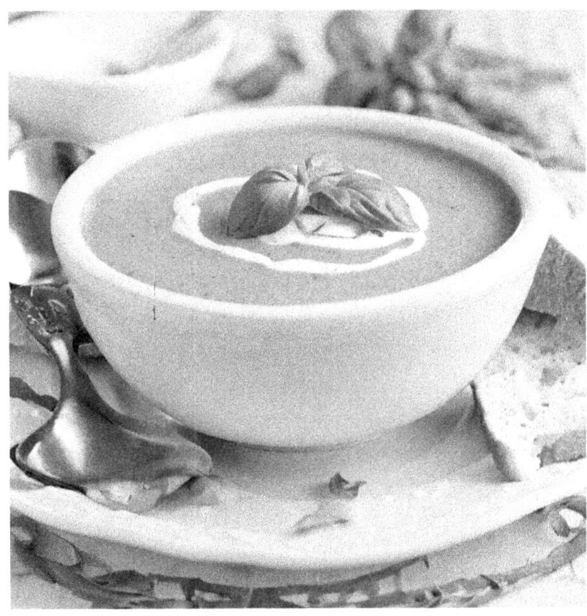

8. Sweet Potato and Leek Soup

Ingredients:

- 2 tablespoons olive oil
- 3 leeks, white and light green parts only, cleaned and sliced
- 2 pounds sweet potatoes, peeled and cubed
- 4 cups vegetable broth
- Salt and pepper to taste
- 1/2 cup heavy cream or coconut milk

Instructions:

1. In a large pot, heat olive oil over medium heat. Add leeks and cook until soft, about 5 minutes.
2. Add sweet potatoes and vegetable broth. Season with salt and pepper. Bring to a boil, then simmer until sweet potatoes are tender, about 20 minutes.
3. Purée the soup in the pot using an immersion blender or transfer to a blender in batches until smooth.
4. Stir in cream or coconut milk and warm through.
5. Serve hot.

Nutrition Info per Serving (serves 6):

- Calories: 250
- Protein: 3g
- Carbohydrates: 37g
- Fat: 10g
- Sodium: 700mg
- Fiber: 5g

Cooking Time: 40 minutes

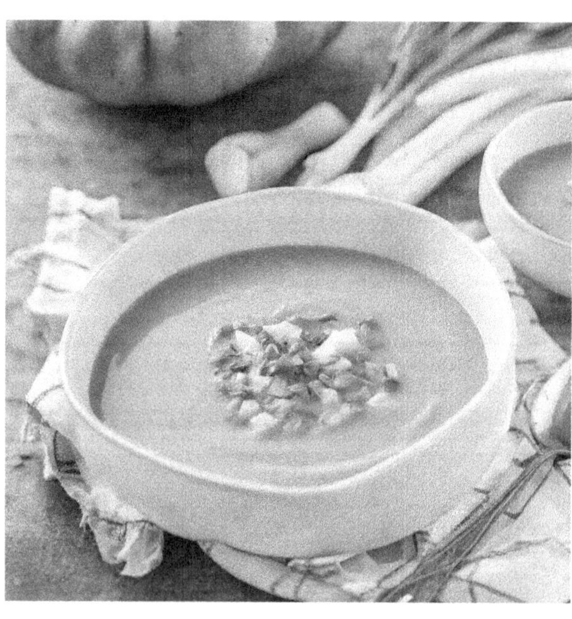

9. Eggplant Parmesan

Ingredients:

- 2 large eggplants, sliced into 1/2-inch thick rounds
- Salt, to draw out moisture from eggplant
- 2 cups marinara sauce
- 2 cups shredded mozzarella cheese
- 1/2 cup grated Parmesan cheese
- 1 cup all-purpose flour, for dredging
- 2 large eggs, beaten
- 2 cups breadcrumbs
- Olive oil, for frying
- Fresh basil for garnish

Instructions:

1. Sprinkle salt on both sides of the eggplant slices and let them sit for 30 minutes to draw out moisture. Pat dry with paper towels.
2. Preheat the oven to 375°F (190°C).
3. Dredge eggplant slices in flour, dip in beaten eggs, and then coat with breadcrumbs.
4. Heat olive oil in a large skillet over medium heat. Fry eggplant slices until golden brown on both sides. Drain on paper towels.
5. Spread a thin layer of marinara sauce on the bottom of a baking dish. Layer eggplant slices, top with more sauce, and sprinkle with mozzarella and Parmesan cheeses. Repeat layers.
6. Bake for 25-30 minutes, until cheese is bubbly and golden. Garnish with fresh basil before serving.

Nutrition Info per Serving (serves 6):

- Calories: 450 Protein: 20g Carbohydrates: 50g Fat: 20g
- Sodium: 900mg
- Fiber: 6g

Cooking Time: 1 hour 10 minutes (including preparation time)

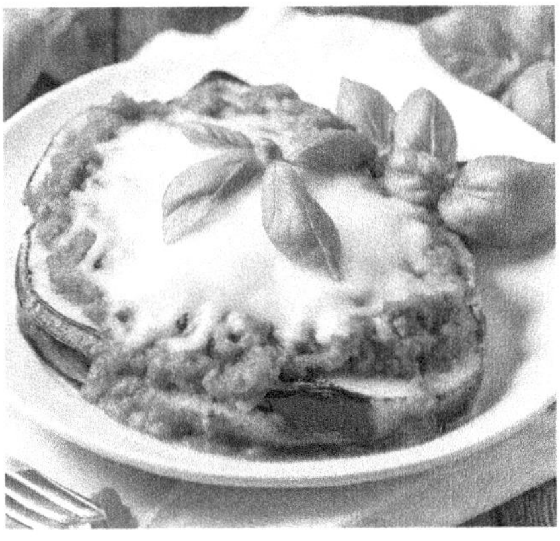

10. Vegetable Lasagna

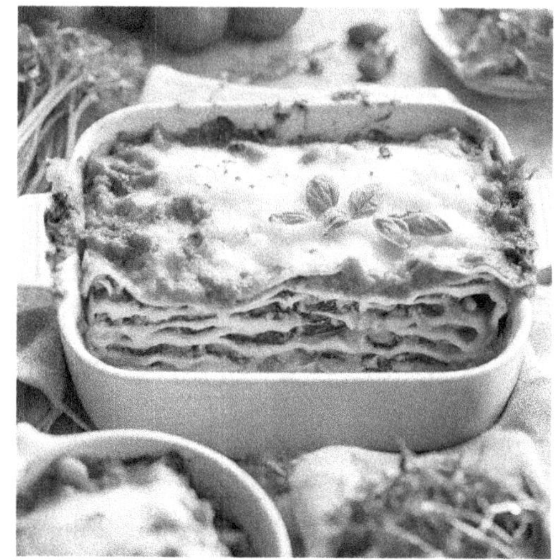

Ingredients:

- 9 lasagna noodles
- 2 tablespoons olive oil
- 1 zucchini, sliced
- 1 bell pepper, chopped
- 1 small eggplant, cubed
- 3 cups spinach
- 2 cups ricotta cheese
- 1 egg
- 3 cups marinara sauce
- 2 cups shredded mozzarella cheese
- 1/2 cup grated Parmesan cheese
- Salt and pepper to taste

Instructions:

1. Cook lasagna noodles according to package instructions. Drain and set aside.
2. In a skillet, heat olive oil over medium heat. Sauté zucchini, bell pepper, and eggplant until softened. Add spinach and cook until wilted. Season with salt and pepper.
3. In a bowl, mix ricotta cheese with the egg.
4. Preheat the oven to 375°F (190°C).
5. Spread a layer of marinara sauce in the bottom of a baking dish. Layer noodles, ricotta mixture, vegetables, mozzarella, and sauce. Repeat layers, ending with mozzarella and Parmesan on top.
6. Cover with foil and bake for 30 minutes. Remove foil and bake for an additional 15 minutes, until cheese is golden.
7. Let cool for 10 minutes before serving.

Nutrition Info per Serving (serves 8):

- Calories: 350
- Protein: 18g
- Carbohydrates: 35g
- Fat: 16g
- Sodium: 700mg
- Fiber: 4g

Cooking Time: 1 hour 15 minutes

11. Creamy Polenta with Roasted Vegetables

Ingredients for Polenta:

- 1 cup polenta
- 4 cups water or vegetable broth
- 1/2 teaspoon salt
- 1/4 cup grated Parmesan cheese
- 2 tablespoons butter

Ingredients for Roasted Vegetables:

- 2 cups mixed vegetables (zucchini, bell peppers, cherry tomatoes)
- 2 tablespoons olive oil
- Salt and pepper to taste

Instructions:

1. Preheat the oven to 425°F (220°C). Toss vegetables with olive oil, salt, and pepper. Spread on a baking sheet and roast for 20-25 minutes, until tender and caramelized.
2. For the polenta, bring water or broth to a boil. Gradually whisk in polenta and salt. Reduce heat to low and cook, stirring frequently, until thickened, about 20 minutes. Stir in Parmesan and butter.
3. Serve roasted vegetables over creamy polenta.

Nutrition Info per Serving (serves 4):

- Calories: 300
- Protein: 8g
- Carbohydrates: 45g
- Fat: 10g
- Sodium: 650mg
- Fiber: 5g

Cooking Time: 45 minutes

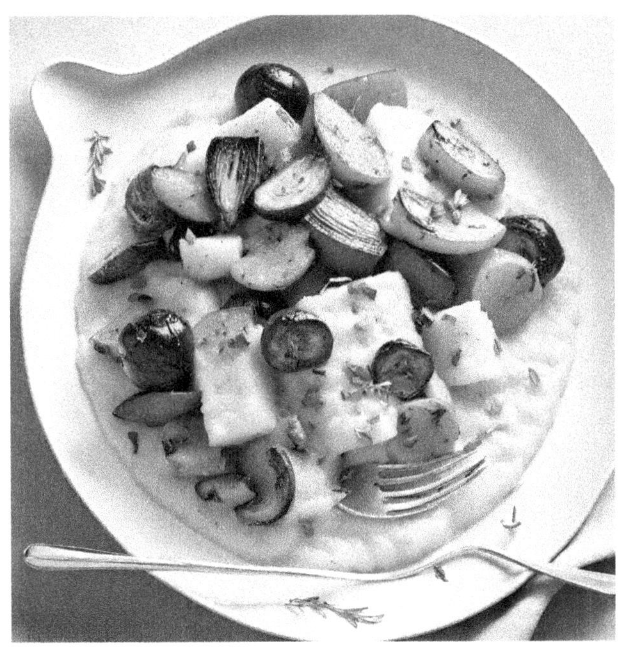

12. Sauteed Green Beans

Ingredients:

- 1 pound green beans, trimmed
- 2 tablespoons olive oil
- 2 cloves garlic, minced
- Salt and pepper to taste
- 1/4 cup water

Instructions:

1. Heat olive oil in a large skillet over medium heat. Add garlic and sauté for 1 minute.
2. Add green beans and water. Cover and cook for 5 minutes.
3. Remove the cover, increase heat to medium-high, and continue cooking until water has evaporated and green beans are tender but still crisp. Season with salt and pepper.
4. Serve immediately.

Nutrition Info per Serving (serves 4):

- Calories: 80
- Protein: 2g
- Carbohydrates: 8g
- Fat: 5g
- Sodium: 10mg
- Fiber: 3g

Cooking Time: 15 minutes

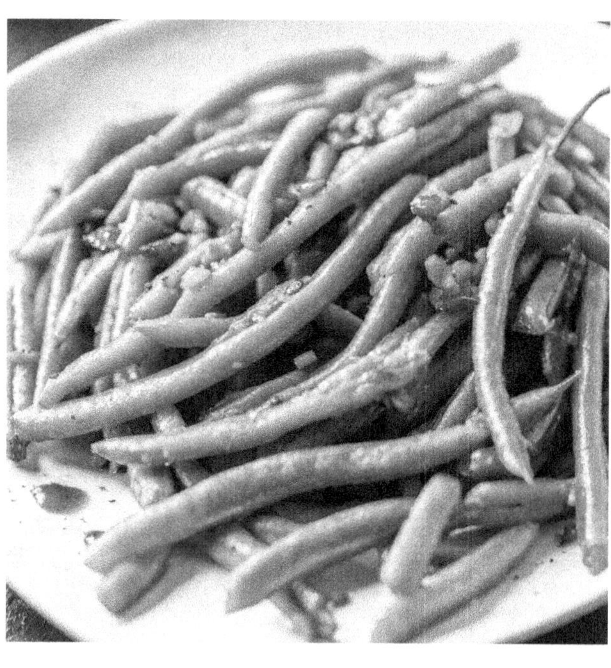

13. Squash Casserole

Ingredients:

- 4 cups sliced yellow squash
- 1/2 cup chopped onion
- 2 eggs, beaten
- 1 cup sour cream
- 1 cup shredded cheddar cheese
- 1 cup breadcrumbs
- 2 tablespoons butter, melted
- Salt and pepper to taste

Instructions:

1. Preheat the oven to 350°F (175°C). Grease a casserole dish.
2. In a large skillet, sauté squash and onion until soft. Drain any excess liquid.
3. In a bowl, mix eggs, sour cream, half of the cheese, salt, and pepper. Stir in squash and onion.
4. Pour mixture into the prepared casserole dish. Top with remaining cheese and breadcrumbs. Drizzle with melted butter.
5. Bake for 30 minutes, until the top is golden and bubbly.
6. Serve warm.

Nutrition Info per Serving (serves 6):

- Calories: 300
- Protein: 10g
- Carbohydrates: 20g
- Fat: 20g
- Sodium: 400mg
- Fiber: 2g

Cooking Time: 45 minutes

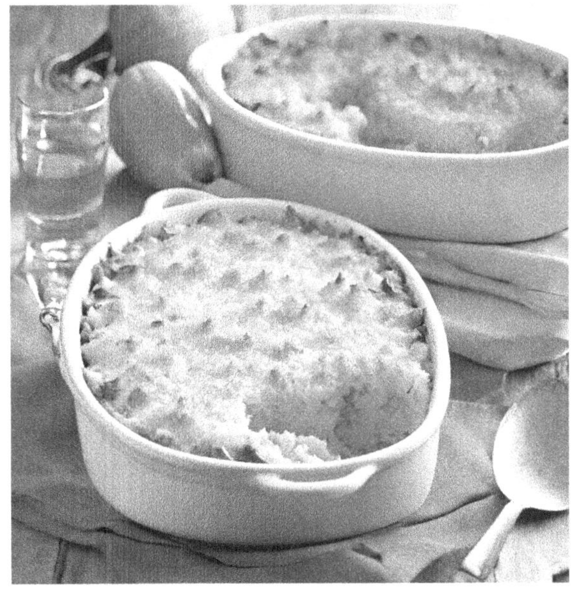

14. Guacamole

Ingredients:

- 3 ripe avocados, peeled and pitted
- Juice of 1 lime
- 1/2 teaspoon salt
- 1/2 cup diced onion
- 3 tablespoons chopped fresh cilantro
- 2 roma tomatoes, diced
- 1 teaspoon minced garlic
- 1 pinch ground cayenne pepper (optional)

Instructions:

1. In a medium bowl, mash together the avocados, lime juice, and salt.
2. Mix in onion, cilantro, tomatoes, and garlic. Stir in cayenne pepper if desired.
3. Serve immediately or cover with plastic wrap directly on the surface and refrigerate to prevent browning.

Nutrition Info per Serving (serves 6):

- Calories: 170
- Protein: 2g
- Carbohydrates: 10g
- Fat: 15g
- Sodium: 200mg
- Fiber: 7g

Cooking Time: 10 minutes

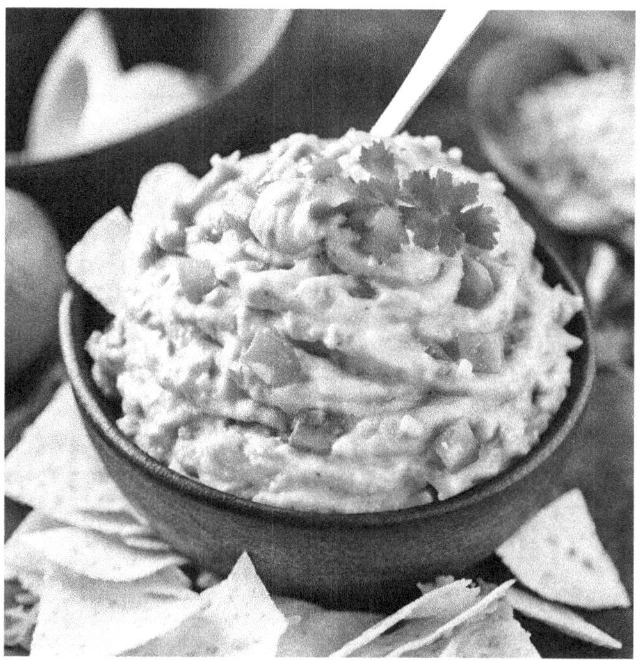

15. Creamy Beet Hummus

Ingredients:

- 1 large beet, roasted and peeled
- 1 can (15 oz) chickpeas, drained and rinsed
- 2 tablespoons tahini
- 2 tablespoons lemon juice
- 1 small garlic clove, minced
- Salt to taste
- 2 tablespoons olive oil

Instructions:

1. In a food processor, blend the roasted beet until smooth.
2. Add chickpeas, tahini, lemon juice, garlic, and salt. Process until smooth.
3. With the processor running, drizzle in olive oil until well incorporated.
4. Serve with vegetables or crackers for dipping.

Nutrition Info per Serving (serves 6):

- Calories: 140
- Protein: 4g
- Carbohydrates: 18g
- Fat: 6g
- Sodium: 300mg
- Fiber: 5g

Cooking Time: 15 minutes (excluding roasting time for beets)

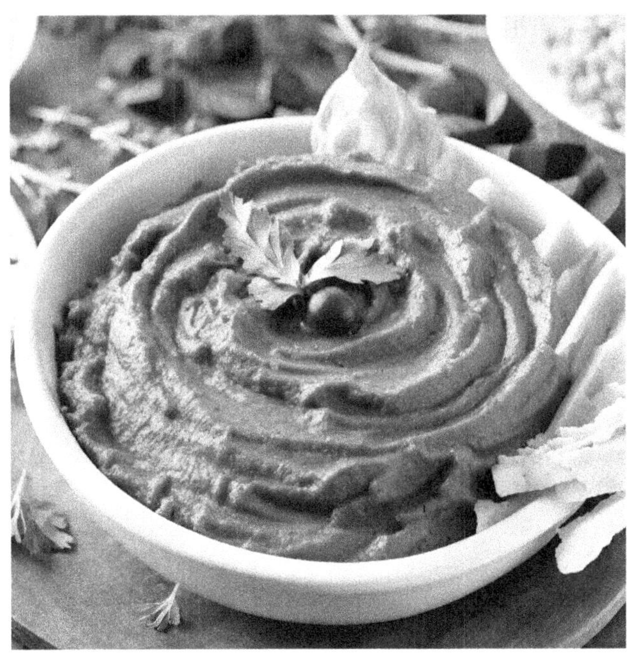

16. Stuffed Mushrooms

Ingredients:

- 12 large mushrooms, stems removed
- 2 tablespoons olive oil
- 1/4 cup finely chopped onion
- 2 cloves garlic, minced
- 1/2 cup breadcrumbs
- 1/4 cup grated Parmesan cheese
- 1/4 cup chopped parsley
- Salt and pepper to taste

Instructions:

1. Preheat the oven to 375°F (190°C).
2. Heat 1 tablespoon olive oil in a skillet over medium heat. Add onion and garlic, and sauté until softened.
3. In a bowl, combine sautéed onion and garlic with breadcrumbs, Parmesan, parsley, salt, and pepper.
4. Stuff each mushroom cap with the mixture. Place on a baking sheet and drizzle with the remaining olive oil.
5. Bake for 20 minutes, until the mushrooms are tender and the tops are golden.
6. Serve warm.

Nutrition Info per Serving (serves 4):

- Calories: 150
- Protein: 5g
- Carbohydrates: 15g
- Fat: 8g
- Sodium: 200mg
- Fiber: 2g

Cooking Time: 30 minutes

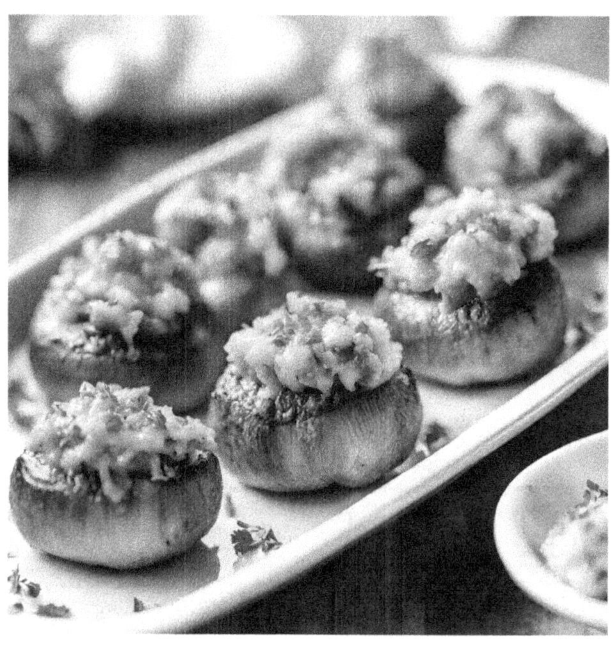

17. Sweet Pea and Avocado Dip

Ingredients:

- 1 cup frozen peas, thawed
- 1 ripe avocado
- Juice of 1 lemon
- 1/4 cup fresh mint leaves
- Salt and pepper to taste
- 1 tablespoon olive oil

Instructions:

1. In a food processor, blend peas, avocado, lemon juice, mint, salt, and pepper until smooth.
2. Drizzle in olive oil while processing to emulsify.
3. Serve chilled with vegetables or crackers for dipping.

Nutrition Info per Serving (serves 4):

- Calories: 160
- Protein: 3g
- Carbohydrates: 12g
- Fat: 12g
- Sodium: 10mg
- Fiber: 6g

Cooking Time: 10 minutes

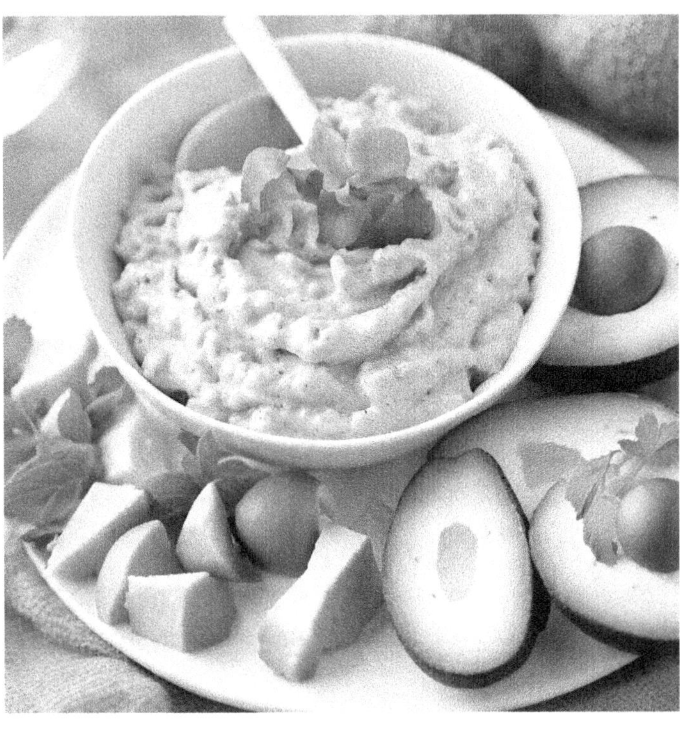

18. Cauliflower Rice

Ingredients:

- 1 head cauliflower, cut into florets
- 2 tablespoons olive oil
- Salt and pepper to taste

Instructions:

1. Pulse cauliflower florets in a food processor until they resemble rice grains.
2. Heat olive oil in a skillet over medium heat. Add cauliflower rice, salt, and pepper.
3. Cook for 5-8 minutes, stirring occasionally, until softened.
4. Serve as a side dish.

Nutrition Info per Serving (serves 4):

- Calories: 80
- Protein: 2g
- Carbohydrates: 8g
- Fat: 5g
- Sodium: 30mg
- Fiber: 4g

Cooking Time: 15 minutes

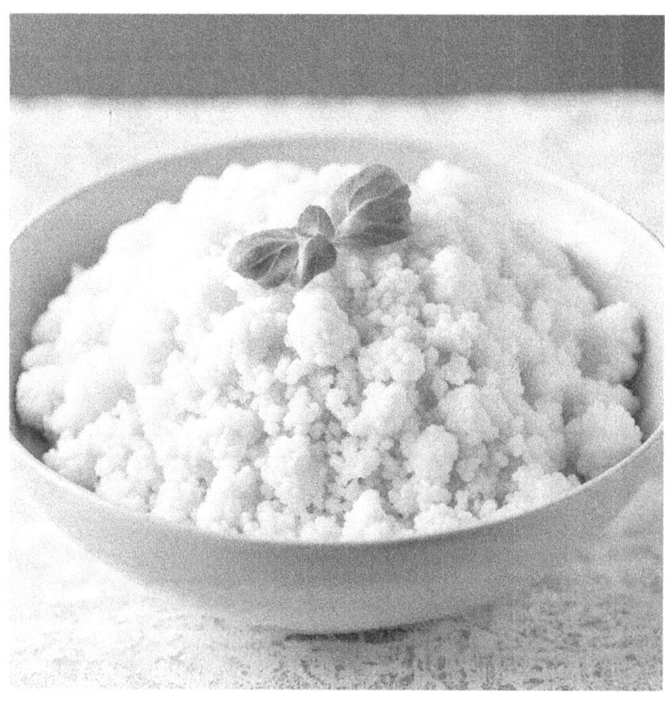

19. Mushroom Stroganoff

Ingredients:

- 1 pound mushrooms, sliced
- 1 large onion, finely chopped
- 2 cloves garlic, minced
- 2 tablespoons olive oil
- 2 tablespoons all-purpose flour
- 1 cup vegetable broth
- 1 cup sour cream or coconut cream
- 2 teaspoons Worcestershire sauce (check for a vegan option if necessary)
- Salt and pepper to taste
- Chopped parsley for garnish
- Cooked egg noodles or rice, for serving

Instructions:

1. In a large skillet, heat the olive oil over medium heat. Add the onion and garlic, sautéing until soft.
2. Add the mushrooms and cook until they release their moisture and start to brown.
3. Sprinkle the flour over the mushrooms and stir to combine. Cook for 1-2 minutes.
4. Gradually add the vegetable broth, stirring constantly, until the mixture thickens.
5. Reduce the heat to low. Stir in the sour cream and Worcestershire sauce. Season with salt and pepper. Heat through, but do not boil.
6. Serve over cooked egg noodles or rice, garnished with parsley.

Nutrition Info per Serving (serves 4):

- Calories: 220 (excluding noodles or rice)
- Protein: 5g
- Carbohydrates: 13g
- Fat: 17g
- Sodium: 300mg
- Fiber: 2g

Cooking Time: 25 minutes

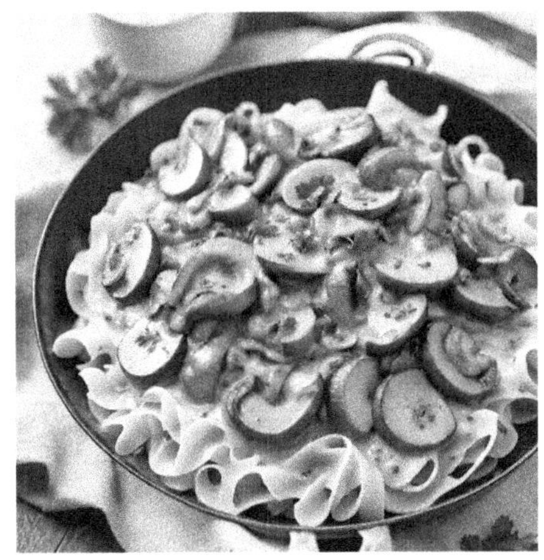

20. Vegetable Minestrone

Ingredients:

- 2 tablespoons olive oil
- 1 onion, chopped
- 2 carrots, chopped
- 2 stalks celery, chopped
- 2 cloves garlic, minced
- 1 zucchini, chopped
- 1 cup green beans, trimmed and cut into 1/2-inch pieces
- 4 cups vegetable broth
- 1 can (14.5 oz) diced tomatoes
- 1 can (15 oz) kidney beans, rinsed and drained
- 1 teaspoon dried oregano
- 1 teaspoon dried basil
- Salt and pepper to taste
- 1 cup small pasta shapes
- Parmesan cheese, for serving (optional)

Instructions:

1. Heat the olive oil in a large pot over medium heat. Add the onion, carrots, celery, and garlic. Cook until the vegetables are softened, about 5 minutes.
2. Add the zucchini and green beans, cooking for another 5 minutes.
3. Stir in the vegetable broth, diced tomatoes with their juice, kidney beans, oregano, basil, salt, and pepper. Bring to a boil.
4. Reduce heat to a simmer and add the pasta. Cook until the pasta is tender, about 10 minutes.
5. Adjust seasoning as needed. Serve hot, garnished with Parmesan cheese if desired.

Nutrition Info per Serving (serves 6):

- Calories: 200
- Protein: 8g
- Carbohydrates: 35g
- Fat: 4g
- Sodium: 700mg
- Fiber: 8g

Cooking Time: 30 minutes

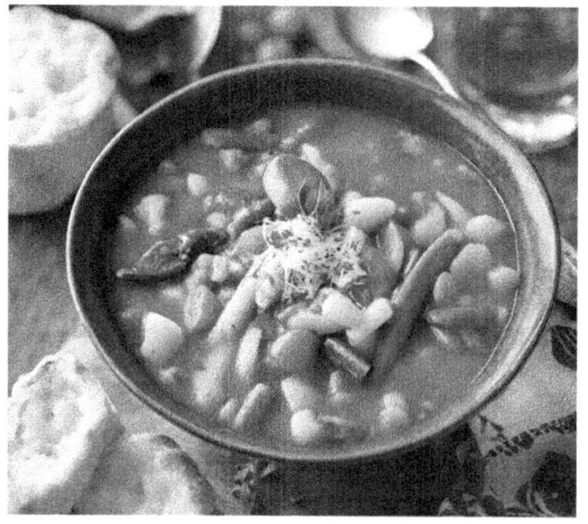

21. Pea and Mint Soup

Ingredients:

- 2 tablespoons olive oil
- 1 onion, chopped
- 2 cups frozen peas
- 4 cups vegetable broth
- 1/4 cup fresh mint leaves
- Salt and pepper to taste
- Sour cream or yogurt, for serving (optional)

Instructions:

1. Heat the olive oil in a large pot over medium heat. Add the onion and cook until soft, about 5 minutes.
2. Add the frozen peas and vegetable broth. Bring to a boil, then reduce heat and simmer for 10 minutes.
3. Remove from heat and add the fresh mint leaves. Using an immersion blender, blend the soup until smooth. Season with salt and pepper to taste.
4. Serve hot, with a dollop of sour cream or yogurt on top if desired.

Nutrition Info per Serving (serves 4):

- Calories: 120
- Protein: 5g
- Carbohydrates: 16g
- Fat: 4g
- Sodium: 950mg
- Fiber: 5g

Cooking Time: 20 minutes

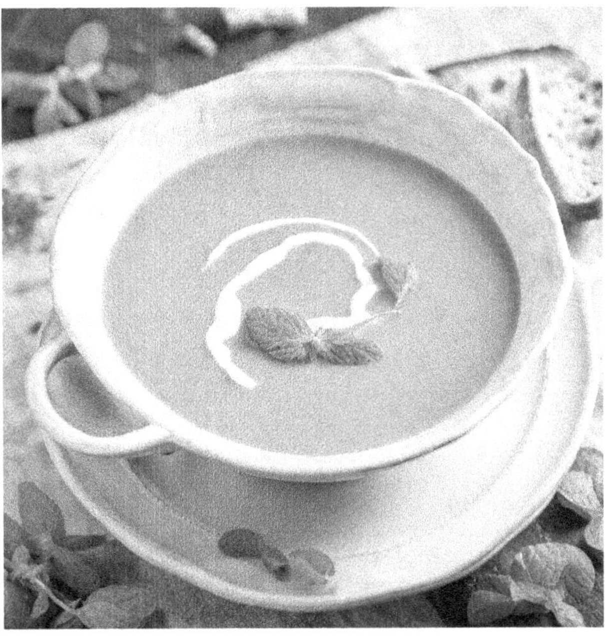

22. Broccoli Slaw

Ingredients:
- 4 cups broccoli slaw mix (shredded broccoli stems, carrots, and red cabbage)
- 1/4 cup mayonnaise
- 2 tablespoons apple cider vinegar
- 1 tablespoon honey or maple syrup
- Salt and pepper to taste
- 1/4 cup sliced almonds, toasted
- 1/4 cup dried cranberries

Instructions:
1. In a large bowl, whisk together mayonnaise, apple cider vinegar, honey, salt, and pepper.
2. Add the broccoli slaw mix to the bowl and toss to coat with the dressing.
3. Refrigerate for at least 30 minutes to allow flavors to meld.
4. Before serving, toss again and top with toasted almonds and dried cranberries.

Nutrition Info per Serving (serves 4):
- Calories: 180
- Protein: 3g
- Carbohydrates: 20g
- Fat: 10g
- Sodium: 200mg
- Fiber: 3g

Cooking Time: 40 minutes (including chilling time)

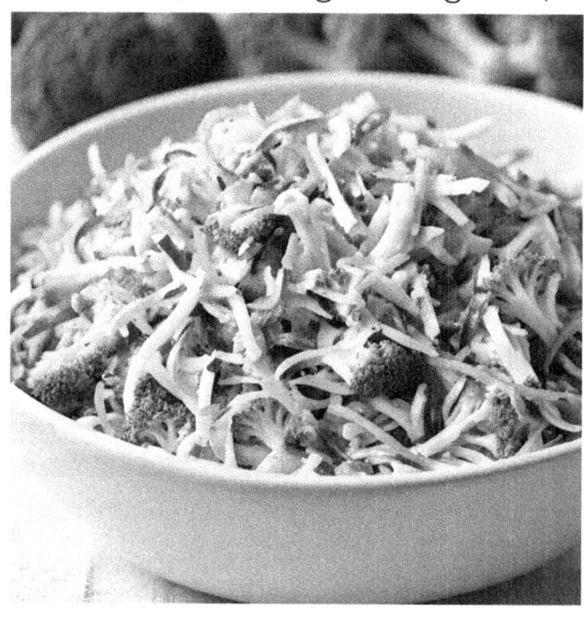

23. Kale and Apple Salad

Ingredients:

- 4 cups kale, stems removed and leaves chopped
- 1 apple, cored and thinly sliced
- 1/4 cup grated Parmesan cheese
- 1/4 cup toasted walnuts, chopped
- 2 tablespoons olive oil
- 1 tablespoon apple cider vinegar
- 1 teaspoon honey
- Salt and pepper to taste

Instructions:

1. In a large bowl, combine the kale, apple slices, Parmesan cheese, and toasted walnuts.
2. In a small bowl, whisk together the olive oil, apple cider vinegar, honey, salt, and pepper.
3. Pour the dressing over the kale mixture and toss until well coated.
4. Let the salad sit for about 10 minutes before serving to allow the kale to soften slightly.

Nutrition Info per Serving (serves 4):

- Calories: 200
- Protein: 6g
- Carbohydrates: 14g
- Fat: 14g
- Sodium: 150mg
- Fiber: 3g

Cooking Time: 20 minutes

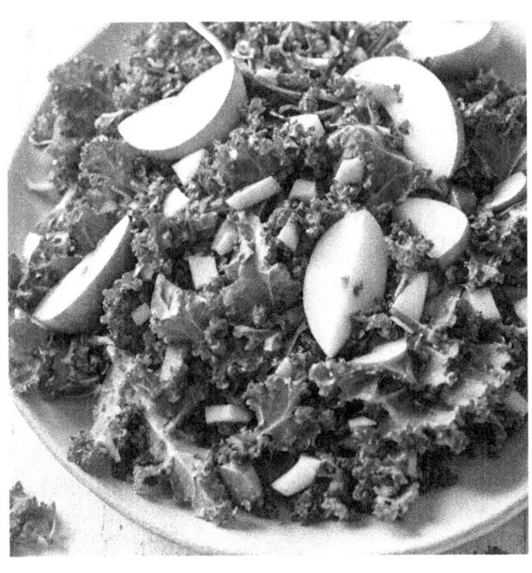

FISH & SEAFOOD RECIPES

1. Honey Garlic Glazed Salmon
Ingredients:
- 4 salmon fillets (6 ounces each)
- Salt and pepper to taste
- 2 tablespoons olive oil
- 3 cloves garlic, minced
- 1/3 cup honey
- 2 tablespoons soy sauce
- 1 tablespoon apple cider vinegar
- Juice of 1 lime

Instructions:
1. Season salmon fillets with salt and pepper.
2. Heat olive oil in a large skillet over medium-high heat. Add salmon fillets, skin side up, and cook for about 4 minutes until golden. Flip the salmon and cook for 2 more minutes.
3. Remove salmon from skillet and set aside. Add garlic to the skillet and sauté until fragrant. Stir in honey, soy sauce, apple cider vinegar, and lime juice. Bring to a simmer.
4. Return the salmon to the skillet, spooning the honey garlic glaze over the fillets. Cook for another 2-3 minutes, until salmon is cooked through and the glaze is thickened.
5. Serve immediately.

Nutrition Info per Serving (serves 4):
- Calories: 350
- Protein: 23g
- Carbohydrates: 24g
- Fat: 18g
- Sodium: 550mg
- Fiber: 0g

Cooking Time: 20 minutes

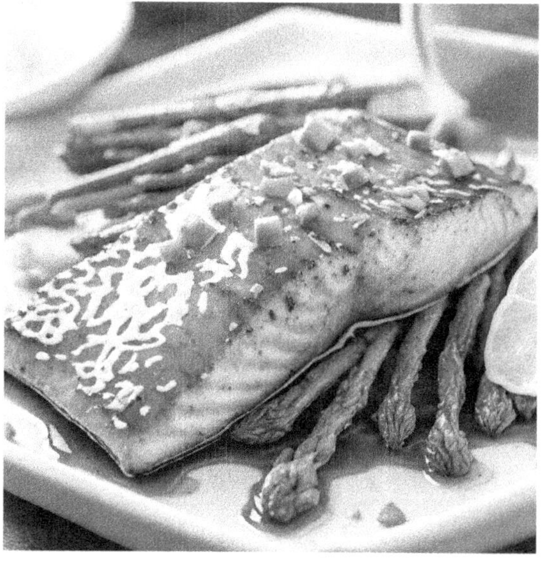

2. Lemon Dill Salmon Patties

Ingredients:

- 2 cans (6 ounces each) salmon, drained and flaked
- 1/2 cup breadcrumbs
- 2 green onions, finely chopped
- 2 tablespoons fresh dill, chopped
- Zest and juice of 1 lemon
- 1 egg, beaten
- Salt and pepper to taste
- 2 tablespoons olive oil for frying

Instructions:

1. In a bowl, combine salmon, breadcrumbs, green onions, dill, lemon zest, lemon juice, and egg. Season with salt and pepper. Mix until well combined.
2. Form the mixture into patties.
3. Heat olive oil in a skillet over medium heat. Fry the patties for about 4 minutes on each side, until golden brown and heated through.
4. Serve hot with a side of salad or your choice of vegetables.

Nutrition Info per Serving (serves 4):

- Calories: 280
- Protein: 22g
- Carbohydrates: 12g
- Fat: 16g
- Sodium: 620mg
- Fiber: 1g

Cooking Time: 20 minutes

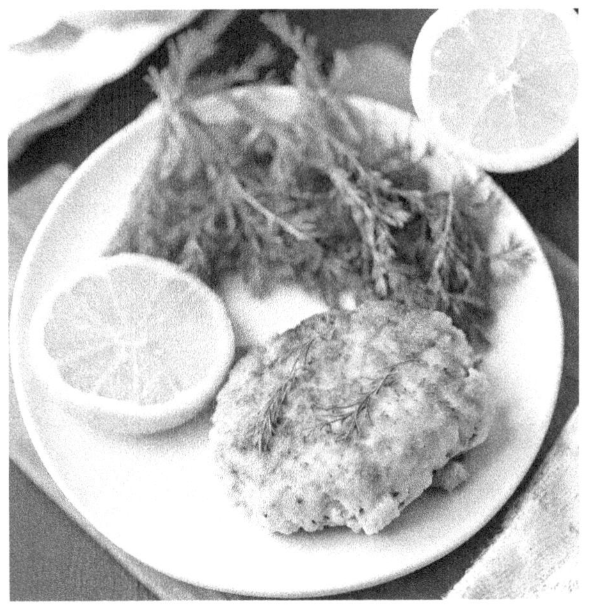

3. Salmon and Spinach Quiche

Ingredients:

- 1 pie crust (store-bought or homemade)
- 1 tablespoon olive oil
- 1 small onion, diced
- 2 cups fresh spinach, chopped
- 4 eggs
- 1 cup heavy cream
- 1 cup cooked salmon, flaked
- 1/2 cup grated Gruyère cheese
- Salt and pepper to taste

Instructions:

1. Preheat the oven to 375°F (190°C). Place the pie crust in a pie dish.
2. Heat olive oil in a skillet over medium heat. Add onion and cook until soft. Add spinach and cook until wilted. Let cool slightly.
3. In a bowl, whisk together eggs and heavy cream. Stir in the cooled spinach mixture, salmon, and Gruyère cheese. Season with salt and pepper.
4. Pour the filling into the pie crust. Bake for 35-40 minutes, until the quiche is set and the crust is golden brown.
5. Let cool for a few minutes before slicing and serving.

Nutrition Info per Serving (serves 6):

- Calories: 390
- Protein: 20g
- Carbohydrates: 18g
- Fat: 27g
- Sodium: 450mg
- Fiber: 1g

Cooking Time: 55 minutes

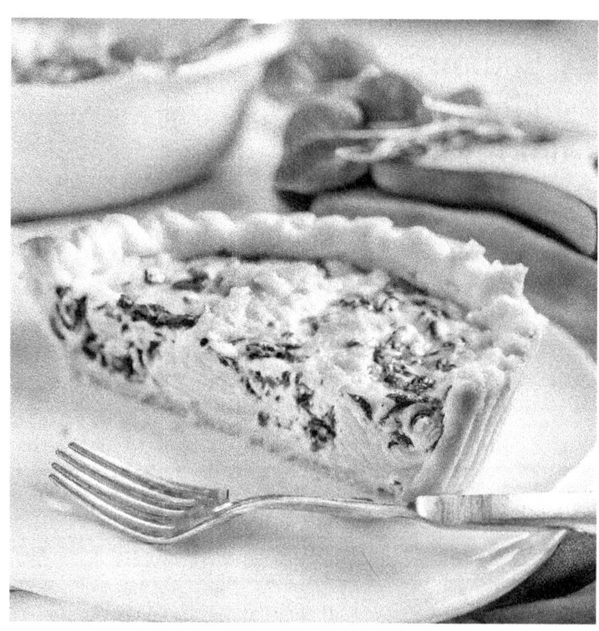

4. Creamy Salmon Pasta

Ingredients:

- 8 ounces pasta (such as fettuccine or penne)
- 2 tablespoons olive oil
- 2 salmon fillets (6 ounces each), cubed
- Salt and pepper to taste
- 1 clove garlic, minced
- 1 cup heavy cream
- 1/2 cup grated Parmesan cheese
- 1 tablespoon fresh dill, chopped
- Zest of 1 lemon

Instructions:

1. Cook pasta according to package instructions. Drain and set aside.
2. Heat olive oil in a skillet over medium heat. Season salmon with salt and pepper and add to the skillet. Cook until salmon is just done, about 4 minutes. Remove salmon and set aside.
3. In the same skillet, add garlic and sauté for 1 minute. Add heavy cream and bring to a simmer. Stir in Parmesan cheese until melted.
4. Add cooked pasta, salmon, dill, and lemon zest to the skillet. Toss to combine and heat through.
5. Serve immediately, garnished with more dill and Parmesan if desired.

Nutrition Info per Serving (serves 4):

- Calories: 600
- Protein: 27g
- Carbohydrates: 45g
- Fat: 34g
- Sodium: 300mg
- Fiber: 2g

Cooking Time: 30 minutes

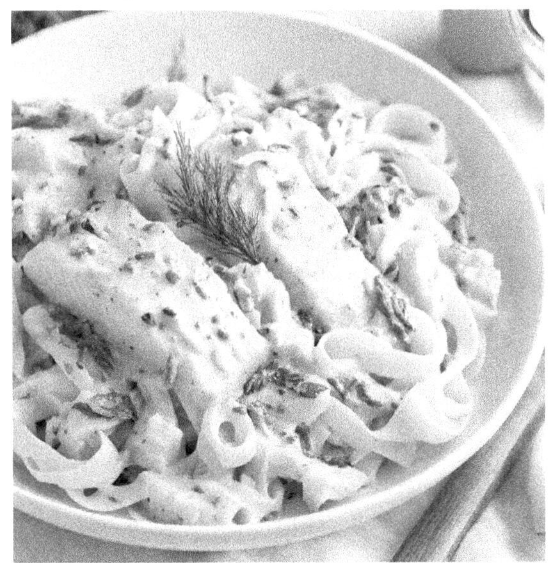

5. Maple Soy Grilled Salmon

Ingredients:

- 4 salmon fillets (6 ounces each)
- 1/4 cup soy sauce
- 1/4 cup maple syrup
- 2 tablespoons olive oil
- 1 garlic clove, minced
- 1 teaspoon ground ginger

Instructions:

1. In a bowl, whisk together soy sauce, maple syrup, olive oil, garlic, and ginger.
2. Place salmon fillets in a shallow dish and pour the marinade over them. Marinate in the refrigerator for at least 30 minutes, up to 2 hours.
3. Preheat the grill to medium-high heat. Remove salmon from marinade, letting excess drip off.
4. Grill salmon for about 5 minutes on each side, or until cooked to your liking.
5. Serve immediately, with extra marinade drizzled over the top if desired.

Nutrition Info per Serving (serves 4):

- Calories: 370
- Protein: 23g
- Carbohydrates: 18g
- Fat: 22g
- Sodium: 880mg
- Fiber: 0g

Cooking Time: 40 minutes (including marinating time)

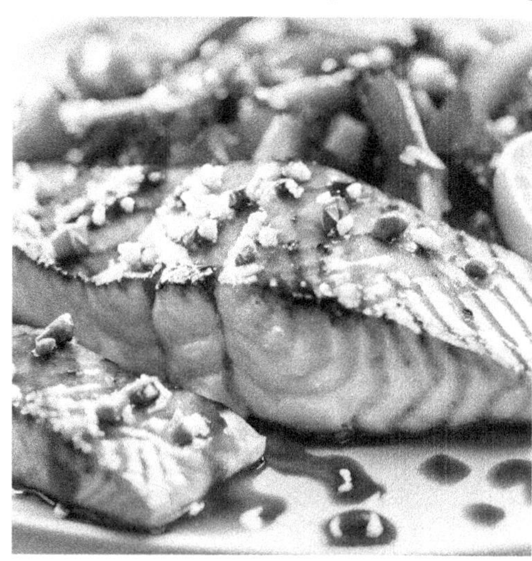

6. Tuna and White Bean Salad

Ingredients:

- 2 cans (5 ounces each) tuna in water, drained
- 1 can (15 ounces) white beans, rinsed and drained
- 1/4 cup red onion, finely chopped
- 2 tablespoons capers, rinsed
- 1/4 cup olive oil
- Juice of 1 lemon
- Salt and pepper to taste
- 2 tablespoons fresh parsley, chopped

Instructions:

1. In a bowl, combine tuna, white beans, red onion, and capers.
2. In a small bowl, whisk together olive oil, lemon juice, salt, and pepper.
3. Pour the dressing over the tuna mixture and toss gently.
4. Garnish with fresh parsley before serving.

Nutrition Info per Serving (serves 4):

- Calories: 290
- Protein: 22g
- Carbohydrates: 23g
- Fat: 13g
- Sodium: 590mg
- Fiber: 6g

Cooking Time: 10 minutes

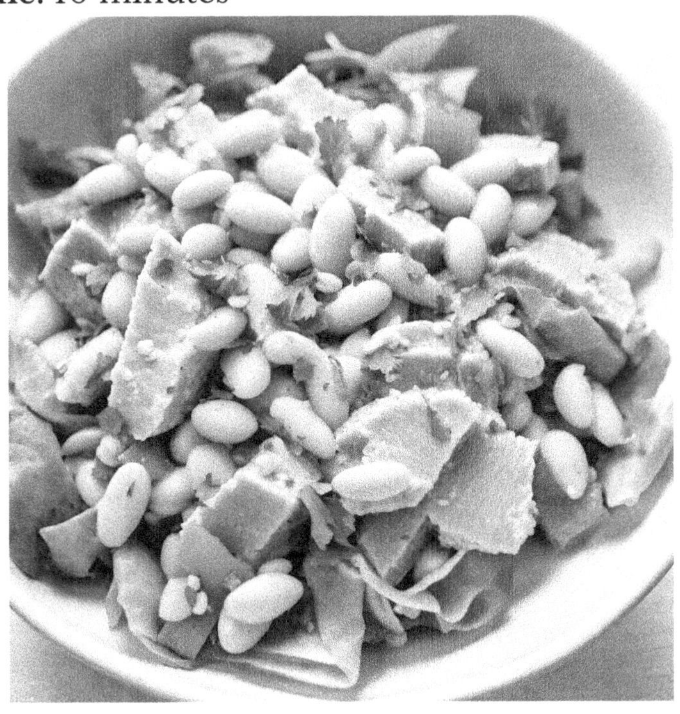

7. Mediterranean Tuna Lettuce Wraps

Ingredients:

- 2 cans (5 ounces each) tuna in olive oil, drained
- 1/2 cup cucumber, diced
- 1/4 cup Kalamata olives, chopped
- 1/4 cup sun-dried tomatoes, chopped
- 1/4 cup feta cheese, crumbled
- 2 tablespoons fresh lemon juice
- 1 tablespoon olive oil
- Salt and pepper to taste
- Romaine lettuce leaves for wrapping

Instructions:

1. In a bowl, combine tuna, cucumber, olives, sun-dried tomatoes, and feta cheese.
2. Drizzle with lemon juice and olive oil. Season with salt and pepper. Toss gently to combine.
3. Spoon the mixture onto romaine lettuce leaves and serve as wraps.

Nutrition Info per Serving (serves 4):

- Calories: 200
- Protein: 18g
- Carbohydrates: 5g
- Fat: 12g
- Sodium: 480mg
- Fiber: 1g

Cooking Time: 15 minutes

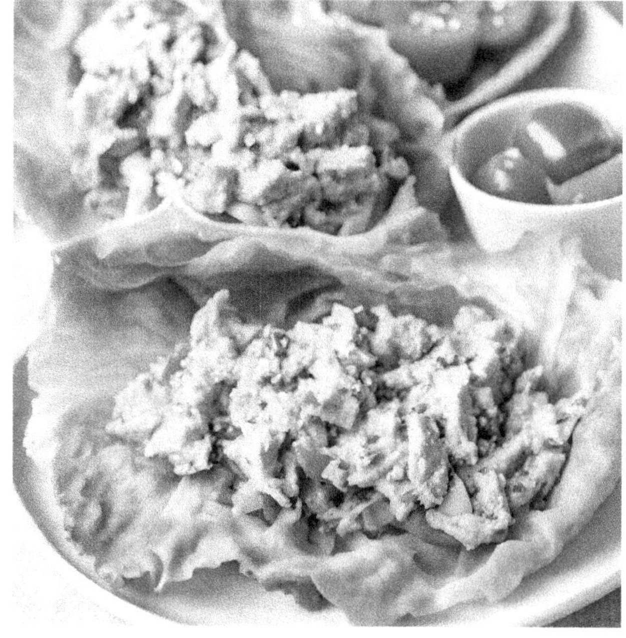

8. Tuna Stuffed Avocados

Ingredients:

- 2 avocados, halved and pitted
- 1 can (5 ounces) tuna in water, drained
- 1/4 cup mayonnaise
- 1/4 cup red bell pepper, diced
- 2 tablespoons red onion, minced
- 1 tablespoon cilantro, chopped
- Juice of 1 lime
- Salt and pepper to taste

Instructions:

1. Scoop out some of the avocado from the halves to create more space for the filling, and chop the scooped avocado.
2. In a bowl, mix the tuna, mayonnaise, red bell pepper, red onion, cilantro, lime juice, and the chopped avocado. Season with salt and pepper.
3. Fill the avocado halves with the tuna mixture.
4. Serve immediately or chill before serving.

Nutrition Info per Serving (serves 4):

- Calories: 300
- Protein: 10g
- Carbohydrates: 9g
- Fat: 26g
- Sodium: 200mg
- Fiber: 7g

Cooking Time: 20 minutes

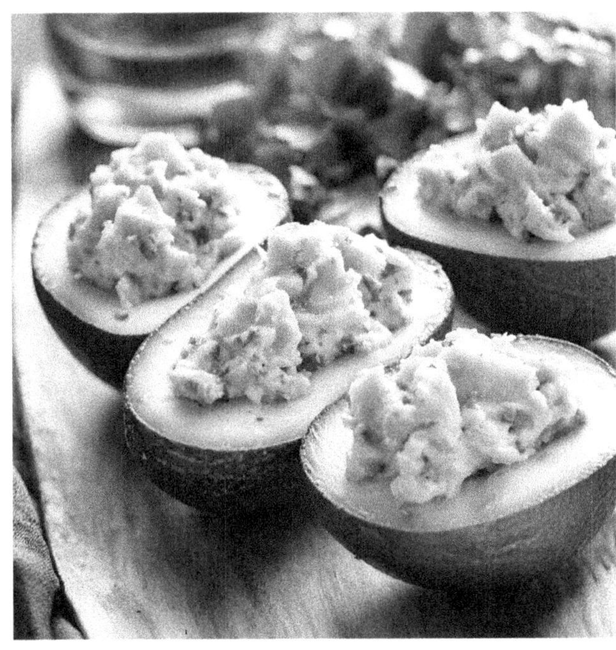

9. Creamy Tuna and Broccoli Pasta Bake

Ingredients:

- 8 ounces pasta (penne or fusilli)
- 1 tablespoon olive oil
- 1 onion, chopped
- 2 cups broccoli florets
- 2 cans (5 ounces each) tuna in water, drained
- 1 cup heavy cream
- 1/2 cup grated Parmesan cheese
- 1/2 cup breadcrumbs
- Salt and pepper to taste

Instructions:

1. Cook pasta according to package instructions, adding broccoli in the last 3 minutes of cooking. Drain and set aside.
2. Preheat the oven to 375°F (190°C). Grease a baking dish.
3. Heat olive oil in a skillet. Add onion and cook until softened.
4. In a large bowl, mix the cooked pasta and broccoli, onion, tuna, heavy cream, and half of the Parmesan cheese. Season with salt and pepper.
5. Transfer the mixture to the prepared baking dish. Top with breadcrumbs and the remaining Parmesan cheese.
6. Bake for 20-25 minutes, until golden and bubbly.
7. Serve warm.

Nutrition Info per Serving (serves 4):

- Calories: 530
- Protein: 27g
- Carbohydrates: 49g
- Fat: 26g
- Sodium: 470mg
- Fiber: 3g

Cooking Time: 45 minutes

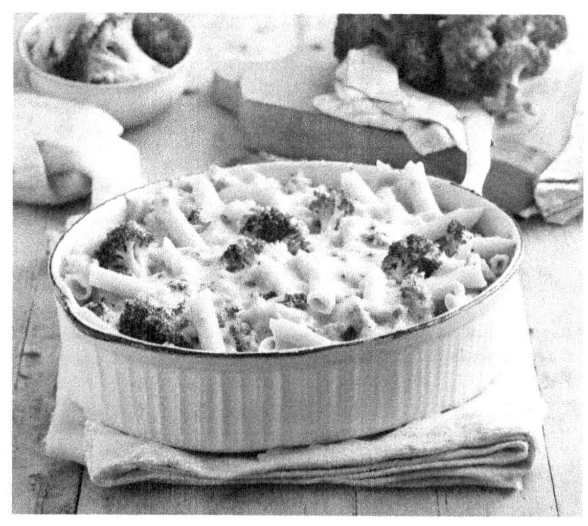

10. Garlic Butter Shrimp

Ingredients:

- 1 pound shrimp, peeled and deveined
- 4 tablespoons butter
- 3 cloves garlic, minced
- Juice of 1 lemon
- 2 tablespoons parsley, chopped
- Salt and pepper to taste

Instructions:

1. Melt butter in a large skillet over medium heat. Add garlic and sauté until fragrant.
2. Add shrimp to the skillet and cook until pink and opaque, about 2-3 minutes per side.
3. Stir in lemon juice and parsley. Season with salt and pepper.
4. Serve immediately, garnished with more parsley if desired.

Nutrition Info per Serving (serves 4):

- Calories: 240
- Protein: 24g
- Carbohydrates: 1g
- Fat: 15g
- Sodium: 880mg
- Fiber: 0g

Cooking Time: 15 minutes

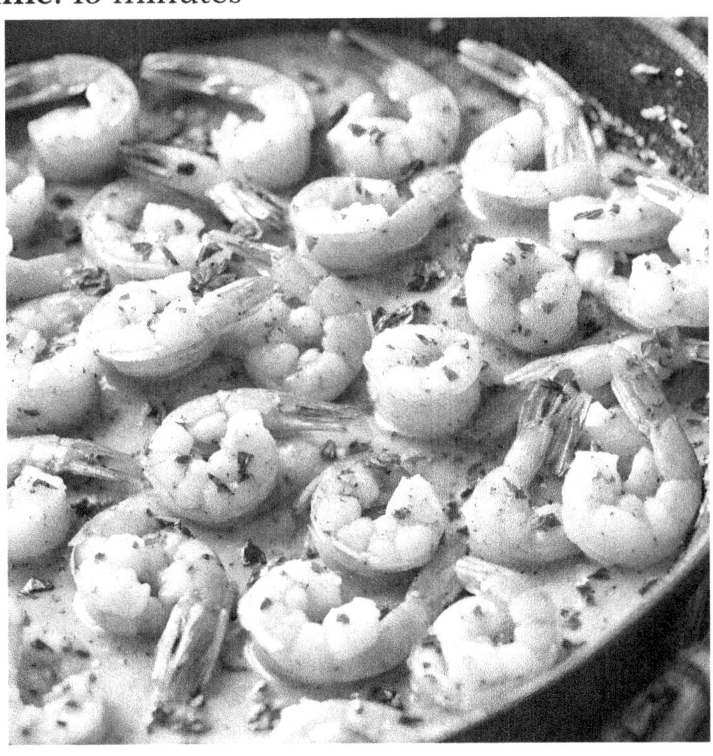

11. Shrimp and Avocado Salad

Ingredients:

- 1 pound cooked shrimp, peeled and deveined
- 2 avocados, diced
- 1/2 cup cherry tomatoes, halved
- 1/4 cup red onion, finely chopped
- 2 tablespoons cilantro, chopped
- Juice of 2 limes
- 2 tablespoons olive oil
- Salt and pepper to taste

Instructions:

1. In a large bowl, combine the shrimp, avocados, cherry tomatoes, red onion, and cilantro.
2. In a small bowl, whisk together lime juice, olive oil, salt, and pepper.
3. Pour the dressing over the salad and gently toss to combine.
4. Serve chilled.

Nutrition Info per Serving (serves 4):

- Calories: 320
- Protein: 25g
- Carbohydrates: 14g
- Fat: 20g
- Sodium: 290mg
- Fiber: 7g

Cooking Time: 15 minutes

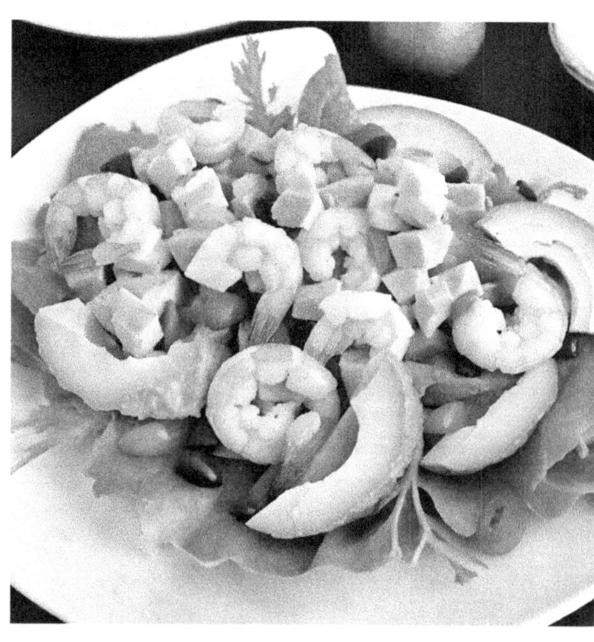

12. Creamy Shrimp Risotto

Ingredients:

- 1 tablespoon olive oil
- 1 small onion, finely chopped
- 1 cup Arborio rice
- 1/2 cup white wine
- 4 cups chicken or vegetable broth, warm
- 1 pound shrimp, peeled and deveined
- 1/2 cup grated Parmesan cheese
- 2 tablespoons butter
- Salt and pepper to taste
- Fresh parsley, chopped for garnish

Instructions:

1. In a large pan, heat olive oil over medium heat. Add onion and cook until translucent.
2. Add Arborio rice, stirring until the grains are well coated and slightly translucent.
3. Pour in white wine, stirring constantly until the wine is absorbed.
4. Add the broth, 1/2 cup at a time, stirring frequently, waiting until it's absorbed before adding more.
5. When the rice is almost done, add the shrimp, cooking until they are pink and opaque.
6. Stir in Parmesan cheese and butter, season with salt and pepper.
7. Garnish with parsley before serving.

Nutrition Info per Serving (serves 4):

- Calories: 510
- Protein: 33g
- Carbohydrates: 51g
- Fat: 18g
- Sodium: 950mg
- Fiber: 2g

Cooking Time: 45 minutes

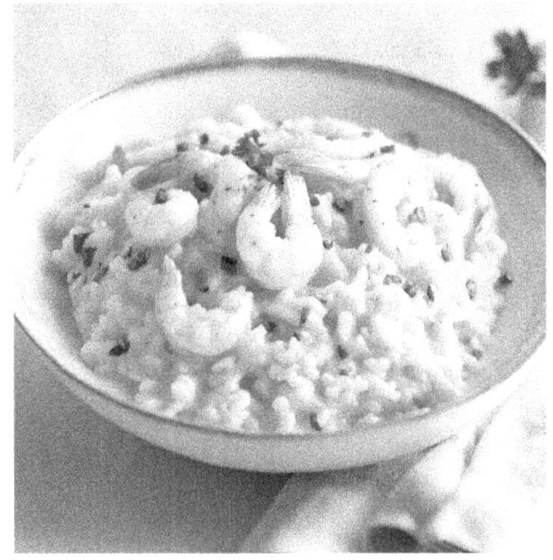

13. Shrimp Scampi with Zoodles

Ingredients:

- 1 pound shrimp, peeled and deveined
- 4 tablespoons butter
- 4 cloves garlic, minced
- 1/2 cup chicken broth or white wine
- Juice of 1 lemon
- 4 medium zucchinis, spiralized into noodles
- Salt and pepper to taste
- Red pepper flakes (optional)
- Fresh parsley, chopped for garnish
- Grated Parmesan cheese for serving

Instructions:

1. Melt butter in a large skillet over medium heat. Add garlic and sauté until fragrant.
2. Add shrimp, cooking until pink and opaque. Remove shrimp from the skillet.
3. Pour chicken broth or white wine into the skillet, adding lemon juice. Simmer until slightly reduced.
4. Add zucchini noodles (zoodles) to the skillet, cooking until tender, about 2-3 minutes.
5. Return shrimp to the skillet. Season with salt, pepper, and red pepper flakes if using. Toss to combine.
6. Garnish with parsley and serve with grated Parmesan cheese.

Nutrition Info per Serving (serves 4):

- Calories: 290
- Protein: 24g
- Carbohydrates: 8g
- Fat: 18g
- Sodium: 710mg
- Fiber: 2g

Cooking Time: 30 minutes

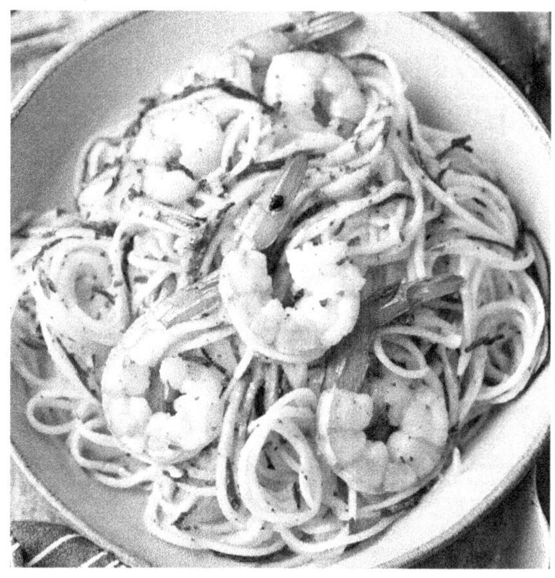

14. Lemon Butter Baked Cod

Ingredients:

- 4 cod fillets (6 ounces each)
- 4 tablespoons butter, melted
- Juice of 1 lemon
- 2 cloves garlic, minced
- 1 teaspoon dried parsley
- Salt and pepper to taste
- Lemon slices for garnish

Instructions:

1. Preheat the oven to 400°F (200°C). Line a baking sheet with parchment paper.
2. Place cod fillets on the prepared baking sheet.
3. In a small bowl, mix together melted butter, lemon juice, garlic, and parsley. Season with salt and pepper.
4. Pour the butter mixture over the cod fillets.
5. Bake for 12-15 minutes, or until the fish flakes easily with a fork.
6. Garnish with lemon slices before serving.

Nutrition Info per Serving (serves 4):

- Calories: 220
- Protein: 23g
- Carbohydrates: 1g
- Fat: 14g
- Sodium: 160mg
- Fiber: 0g

Cooking Time: 20 minutes

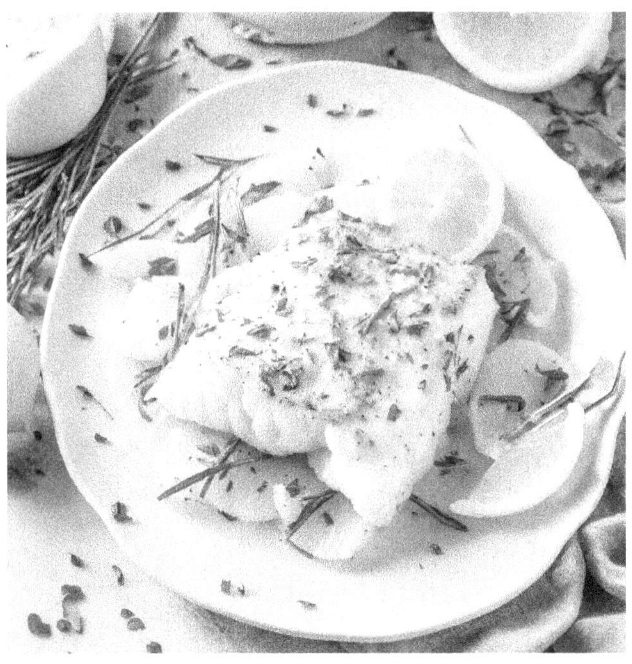

15. Fish Pie with Sweet Potato Topping

Ingredients:

- 1 pound mixed fish fillets (cod, salmon, haddock), cubed
- 1 cup milk
- 1 bay leaf
- 2 tablespoons butter
- 2 tablespoons flour
- 1/2 cup frozen peas
- 1/2 cup corn
- 2 large sweet potatoes, peeled and cubed
- 2 tablespoons olive oil
- Salt and pepper to taste
- Fresh parsley, chopped for garnish

Instructions:

1. Preheat the oven to 375°F (190°C).
2. In a saucepan, poach the fish in milk with a bay leaf until just cooked. Remove fish and set aside, reserving the milk.
3. In the same pan, melt butter over medium heat. Stir in flour to make a roux. Gradually add reserved milk, whisking until thickened. Stir in peas and corn. Gently fold in the poached fish. Season with salt and pepper.
4. Transfer the mixture to a baking dish.
5. Boil sweet potatoes until tender. Mash with olive oil, salt, and pepper until smooth.
6. Spread the mashed sweet potatoes over the fish mixture.
7. Bake for 25-30 minutes, until the topping is golden.
8. Garnish with parsley before serving.

Nutrition Info per Serving (serves 4):

- Calories: 450
- Protein: 25g
- Carbohydrates: 35g
- Fat: 23g
- Sodium: 300mg
- Fiber: 5g

Cooking Time: 1 hour

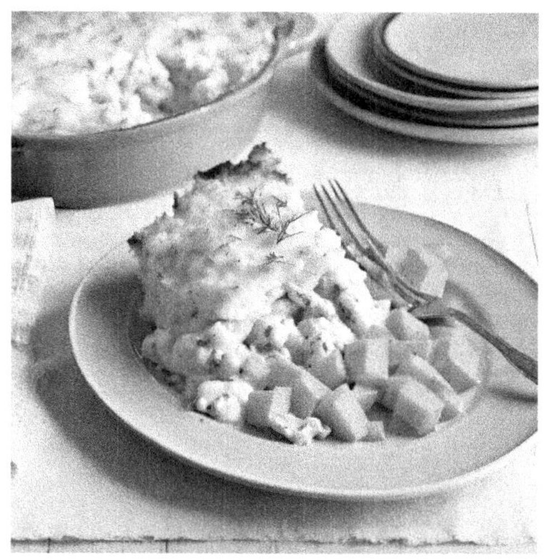

16. Creamy Fish Chowder

Ingredients:

- 2 tablespoons butter
- 1 onion, chopped
- 2 celery stalks, chopped
- 2 carrots, peeled and diced
- 2 potatoes, peeled and cubed
- 4 cups fish or vegetable stock
- 1 pound white fish fillets (e.g., cod, haddock), cut into chunks
- 1 cup heavy cream
- Salt and pepper to taste
- Fresh parsley, chopped for garnish

Instructions:

1. In a large pot, melt butter over medium heat. Add onion, celery, and carrots. Cook until softened, about 5 minutes.
2. Add potatoes and stock. Bring to a boil, then reduce heat and simmer until potatoes are tender, about 15 minutes.
3. Add fish chunks to the pot and cook until opaque and flaky, about 5-7 minutes.
4. Stir in heavy cream and season with salt and pepper. Heat through without boiling.
5. Garnish with fresh parsley before serving.

Nutrition Info per Serving (serves 4):

- Calories: 400
- Protein: 25g
- Carbohydrates: 28g
- Fat: 22g
- Sodium: 950mg
- Fiber: 3g

Cooking Time: 40 minutes

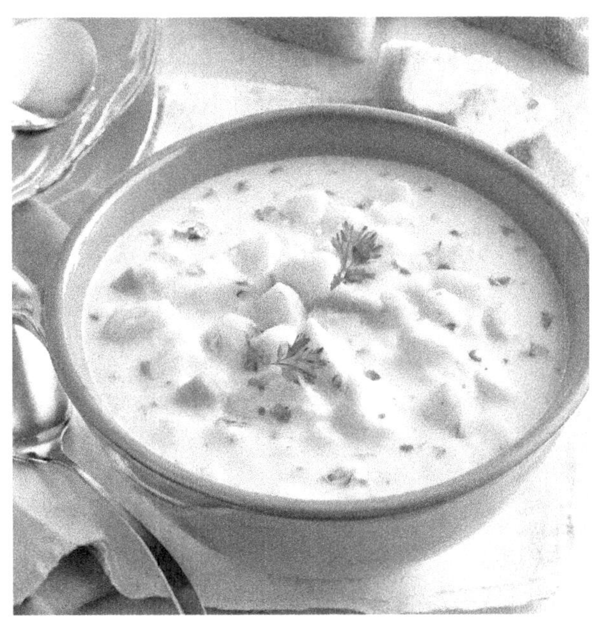

17. Mussels in White Wine Sauce

Ingredients:

- 2 pounds mussels, cleaned and debearded
- 2 tablespoons olive oil
- 4 garlic cloves, minced
- 1 shallot, finely chopped
- 1 cup white wine
- 2 tablespoons butter
- Fresh parsley, chopped for garnish
- Lemon wedges for serving

Instructions:

1. In a large pot, heat olive oil over medium heat. Add garlic and shallot, and sauté until soft.
2. Pour in white wine and bring to a simmer.
3. Add mussels to the pot, cover, and cook until they open, about 5-7 minutes. Discard any that do not open.
4. Stir in butter until melted. Garnish with fresh parsley.
5. Serve hot with lemon wedges on the side.

Nutrition Info per Serving (serves 4):

- Calories: 290
- Protein: 20g
- Carbohydrates: 8g
- Fat: 16g
- Sodium: 480mg
- Fiber: 0g

Cooking Time: 20 minutes

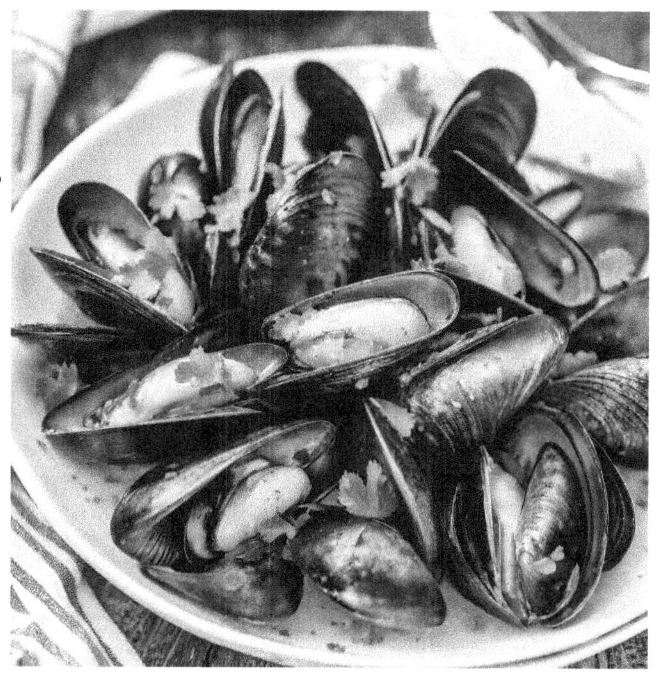

18. Crab Cakes with Remoulade Sauce

Ingredients for Crab Cakes:

- 1 pound lump crab meat, picked over for shells
- 1/2 cup breadcrumbs
- 1/4 cup mayonnaise
- 1 egg, lightly beaten
- 2 teaspoons Dijon mustard
- 2 tablespoons green onions, chopped
- 1 teaspoon Old Bay seasoning
- 2 tablespoons olive oil for frying

Ingredients for Remoulade Sauce:

- 1/2 cup mayonnaise
- 1 tablespoon Dijon mustard
- 1 tablespoon capers, chopped
- 1 tablespoon pickle relish
- 1 teaspoon lemon juice
- 1 teaspoon paprika
- Salt and pepper to taste

Instructions:

1. In a bowl, mix crab meat, breadcrumbs, mayonnaise, egg, Dijon mustard, green onions, and Old Bay seasoning.
2. Form mixture into patties.
3. Heat olive oil in a skillet over medium heat. Fry crab cakes until golden brown on both sides, about 4 minutes per side.
4. For the remoulade sauce, whisk together all ingredients until smooth.
5. Serve crab cakes with remoulade sauce on the side.

Nutrition Info per Serving (serves 4):

- Calories: 370
- Protein: 24g
- Carbohydrates: 14g
- Fat: 24g
- Sodium: 880mg
- Fiber: 1g

Cooking Time: 30 minutes

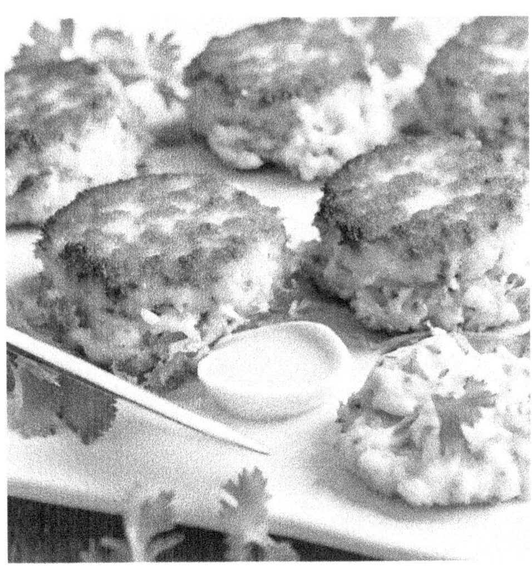

19. Scallop Pasta with Lemon Sauce

Ingredients:

- 8 ounces pasta (linguine or spaghetti)
- 1 pound scallops
- Salt and pepper to taste
- 2 tablespoons butter
- 2 cloves garlic, minced
- Zest and juice of 1 lemon
- 1/2 cup heavy cream
- 1/4 cup grated Parmesan cheese
- Fresh parsley, chopped for garnish

Instructions:

1. Cook pasta according to package instructions. Drain and set aside.
2. Season scallops with salt and pepper. Heat butter in a skillet over medium-high heat. Add scallops and sear until golden brown on both sides, about 2 minutes per side. Remove scallops from skillet.
3. In the same skillet, add garlic and lemon zest. Sauté for 1 minute. Add lemon juice and heavy cream. Bring to a simmer.
4. Stir in cooked pasta and Parmesan cheese. Toss until the pasta is coated in the sauce.
5. Return scallops to the skillet, warming through.
6. Garnish with fresh parsley before serving.

Nutrition Info per Serving (serves 4):

- Calories: 510
- Protein: 28g
- Carbohydrates: 50g
- Fat: 22g
- Sodium: 670mg
- Fiber: 2g

Cooking Time: 30 minutes

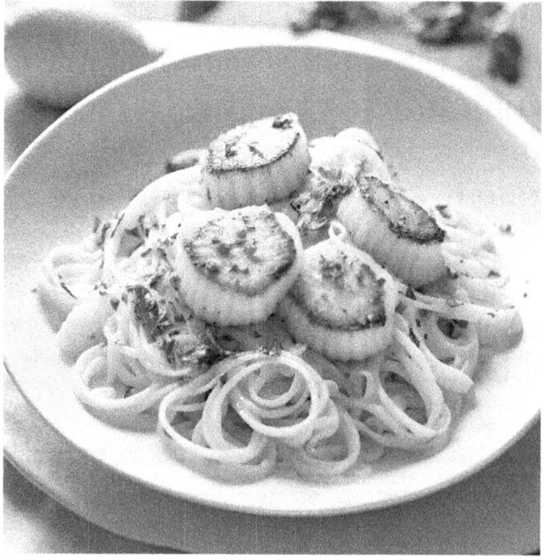

20. Seafood Alfredo

Ingredients:
- 8 ounces fettuccine pasta
- 1 tablespoon olive oil
- 1 cup mixed seafood (shrimp, scallops, and crab meat)
- 2 cloves garlic, minced
- 1 cup heavy cream
- 1/2 cup grated Parmesan cheese
- Salt and pepper to taste
- Fresh parsley, chopped for garnish

Instructions:
1. Cook fettuccine according to package instructions. Drain and set aside.
2. Heat olive oil in a skillet over medium heat. Add mixed seafood and garlic, cooking until seafood is cooked through.
3. Lower the heat and add heavy cream, stirring continuously until it begins to thicken.
4. Stir in Parmesan cheese until melted and the sauce is smooth. Season with salt and pepper.
5. Toss cooked pasta with the Alfredo sauce and seafood. Serve garnished with fresh parsley.

Nutrition Info per Serving (serves 4):
- Calories: 550
- Protein: 25g
- Carbohydrates: 45g
- Fat: 30g
- Sodium: 500mg
- Fiber: 2g

Cooking Time: 30 minutes

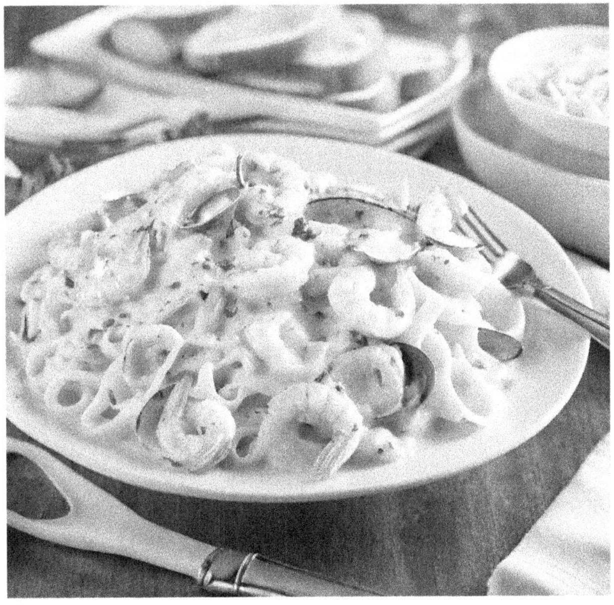

21. Grilled Seafood Platter

Ingredients:

- 4 large shrimp, peeled and deveined
- 4 sea scallops
- 2 salmon fillets, 4 ounces each
- 2 tablespoons olive oil
- Salt and pepper to taste
- Lemon wedges for serving
- Fresh herbs for garnish (dill, parsley)

Instructions:

1. Preheat grill to medium-high heat.
2. Brush seafood with olive oil and season with salt and pepper.
3. Grill shrimp, scallops, and salmon, turning once, until cooked through - about 3-4 minutes per side for shrimp and scallops, 5-6 minutes per side for salmon.
4. Serve the grilled seafood on a platter with lemon wedges and garnish with fresh herbs.

Nutrition Info per Serving (serves 4):

- Calories: 300
- Protein: 28g
- Carbohydrates: 1g
- Fat: 20g
- Sodium: 220mg
- Fiber: 0g

Cooking Time: 20 minutes

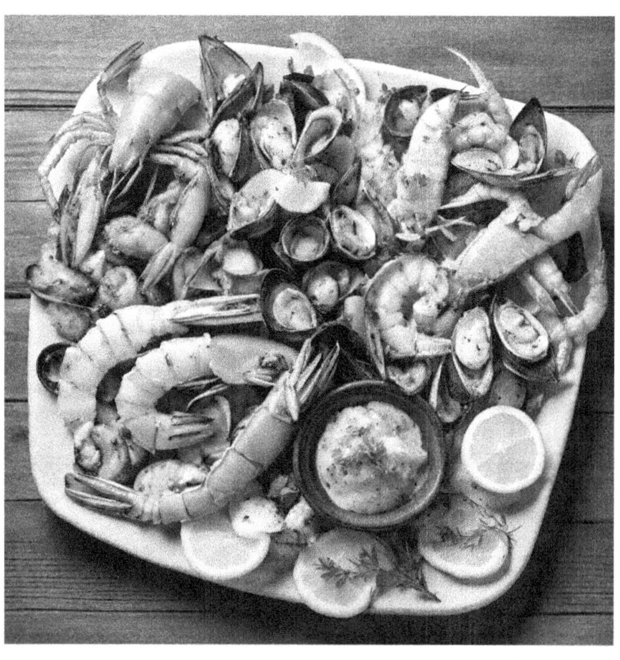

22. Seafood Salad with Citrus Vinaigrette

Ingredients:

- 2 cups mixed greens
- 1/2 pound cooked mixed seafood (shrimp, crab meat, scallops)
- 1 orange, segmented
- 1/2 avocado, sliced
- 1/4 cup sliced red onion
- **For the Citrus Vinaigrette:**
    - Juice of 1 lemon
    - Juice of 1 orange
    - 2 tablespoons olive oil
    - 1 teaspoon honey
    - Salt and pepper to taste

Instructions:

1. In a large bowl, combine mixed greens, seafood, orange segments, avocado slices, and red onion.
2. In a small bowl, whisk together lemon juice, orange juice, olive oil, honey, salt, and pepper to create the vinaigrette.
3. Drizzle the vinaigrette over the salad and toss gently to combine.
4. Serve immediately.

Nutrition Info per Serving (serves 4):

- Calories: 250
- Protein: 15g
- Carbohydrates: 12g
- Fat: 16g
- Sodium: 150mg
- Fiber: 3g

Cooking Time: 15 minutes

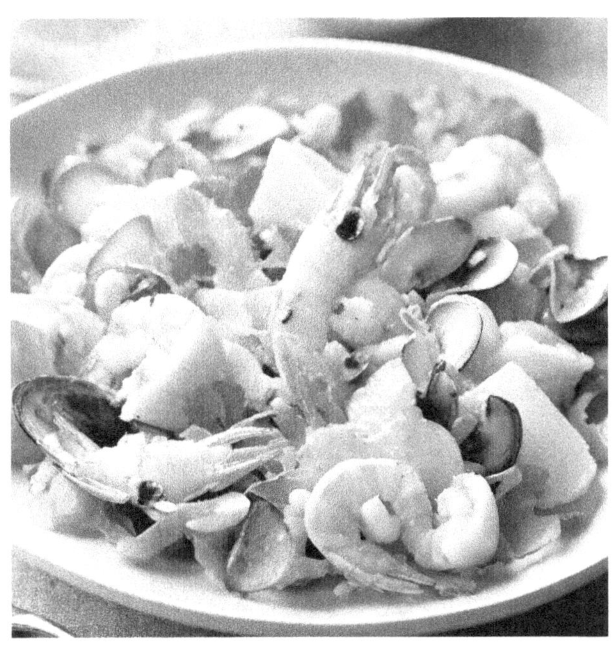

23. Octopus Salad with Lemon and Olive Oil

Ingredients:

- 1 pound cooked octopus, sliced
- 2 tablespoons olive oil
- Juice of 1 lemon
- 1/4 cup chopped parsley
- 1 clove garlic, minced
- Salt and pepper to taste
- Mixed greens for serving

Instructions:

1. In a bowl, combine sliced octopus, olive oil, lemon juice, parsley, and garlic. Season with salt and pepper.
2. Let the salad marinate in the refrigerator for at least 30 minutes.
3. Serve over mixed greens.

Nutrition Info per Serving (serves 4):

- Calories: 180
- Protein: 25g
- Carbohydrates: 4g
- Fat: 7g
- Sodium: 700mg
- Fiber: 0g

Cooking Time: 40 minutes (including marinating time)

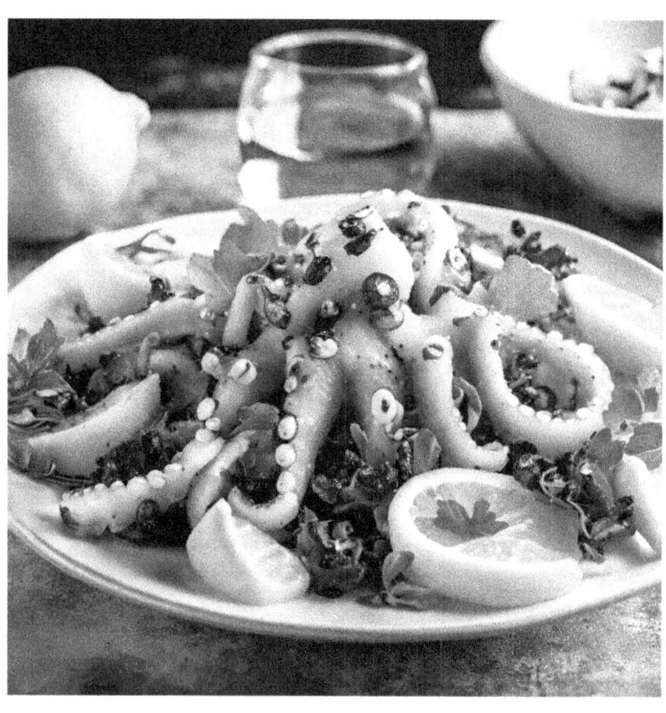

24. Sea Bass with Mediterranean Salsa

Ingredients:

- 4 sea bass fillets, 6 ounces each
- 2 tablespoons olive oil
- Salt and pepper to taste
- **For the Salsa:**
  - 1 cup cherry tomatoes, quartered
  - 1/4 cup Kalamata olives, pitted and chopped
  - 1/4 cup feta cheese, crumbled
  - 2 tablespoons red onion, finely chopped
  - 2 tablespoons fresh basil, chopped
  - Juice of 1 lemon
  - 1 tablespoon olive oil

Instructions:

1. Preheat oven to 400°F (200°C).
2. Place sea bass fillets on a baking sheet. Brush with olive oil and season with salt and pepper.
3. Bake for 12-15 minutes, until fish flakes easily with a fork.
4. While the fish is baking, mix together all salsa ingredients in a bowl.
5. Serve the sea bass topped with Mediterranean salsa.

Nutrition Info per Serving (serves 4):

- Calories: 300
- Protein: 35g
- Carbohydrates: 5g
- Fat: 16g
- Sodium: 350mg
- Fiber: 1g

Cooking Time: 30 minutes

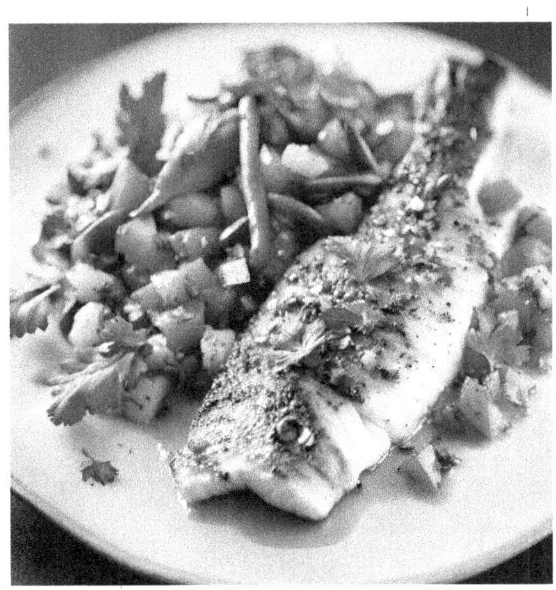

25. Salmon Broth with Noodles

Ingredients:

- 4 cups chicken or vegetable broth
- 1 pound salmon fillet, cut into chunks
- 2 cups noodles (e.g., udon or rice noodles)
- 1 cup spinach leaves
- 1/2 cup sliced mushrooms
- 2 tablespoons soy sauce
- 1 tablespoon ginger, grated
- 2 green onions, sliced
- Salt and pepper to taste

Instructions:

1. In a large pot, bring broth to a boil. Add ginger and soy sauce.
2. Add noodles to the pot and cook according to package instructions.
3. Add salmon chunks, spinach, and mushrooms in the last 5 minutes of cooking.
4. Season with salt and pepper. Garnish with green onions before serving.

Nutrition Info per Serving (serves 4):

- Calories: 350
- Protein: 25g
- Carbohydrates: 35g
- Fat: 12g
- Sodium: 800mg
- Fiber: 2g

Cooking Time: 25 minutes

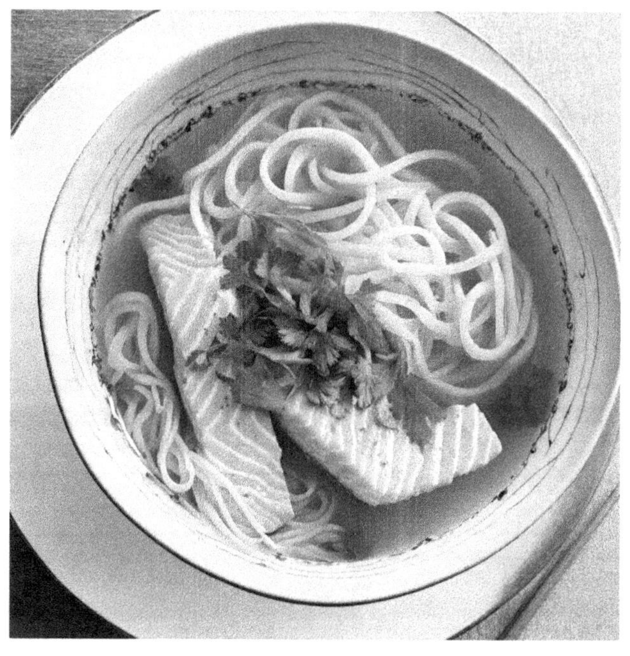

26. Baked Haddock with Olive Tapenade

Ingredients:

- 4 haddock fillets, 6 ounces each
- 2 tablespoons olive oil
- Salt and pepper to taste
- **For the Olive Tapenade:**
    - 1/2 cup pitted Kalamata olives
    - 1 tablespoon capers
    - 2 cloves garlic
    - 2 tablespoons olive oil
    - Juice of 1 lemon

Instructions:

1. Preheat oven to 400°F (200°C). Line a baking sheet with parchment paper.
2. Place haddock fillets on the prepared baking sheet. Brush with olive oil and season with salt and pepper.
3. Bake for 12-15 minutes, until fish flakes easily with a fork.
4. For the tapenade, blend olives, capers, garlic, olive oil, and lemon juice in a food processor until smooth.
5. Serve the haddock topped with olive tapenade.

Nutrition Info per Serving (serves 4):

- Calories: 290
- Protein: 27g
- Carbohydrates: 3g
- Fat: 19g
- Sodium: 610mg
- Fiber: 1g

Cooking Time: 30 minutes

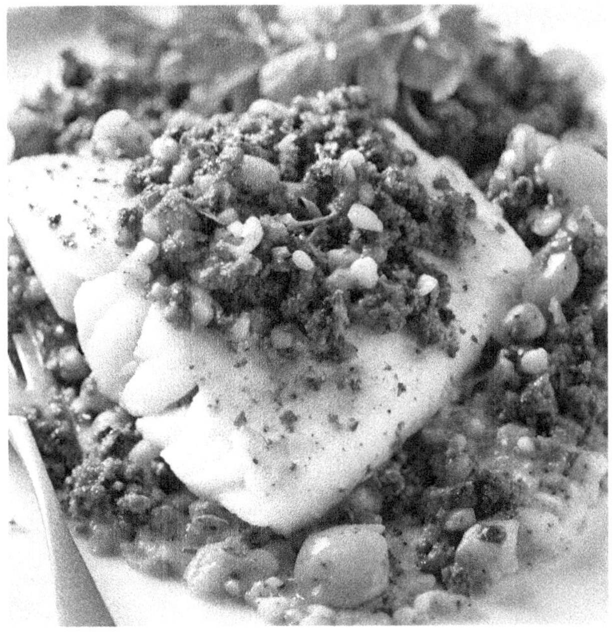

SOUP & STEW RECIPES

1. Mexican Chicken Pozole

Ingredients:

- 2 tablespoons olive oil
- 1 onion, chopped
- 2 cloves garlic, minced
- 1 pound boneless, skinless chicken breasts, cut into bite-size pieces
- 1 teaspoon dried oregano
- 1 teaspoon cumin
- 4 cups chicken broth
- 1 can (15 oz) hominy, drained and rinsed
- 1 can (14.5 oz) diced tomatoes
- Salt and pepper to taste
- Fresh cilantro, diced radishes, and lime wedges for garnish

Instructions:

1. Heat olive oil in a large pot over medium heat. Add onion and garlic, and sauté until softened.
2. Add chicken, oregano, and cumin, cooking until chicken is browned.
3. Stir in chicken broth, hominy, and diced tomatoes. Season with salt and pepper.
4. Bring to a boil, then reduce heat and simmer for 20 minutes.
5. Serve hot, garnished with cilantro, radishes, and lime wedges.

Nutrition Info per Serving (serves 6):

- Calories: 180
- Protein: 20g
- Carbohydrates: 15g
- Fat: 5g
- Sodium: 800mg
- Fiber: 3g

Cooking Time: 40 minutes

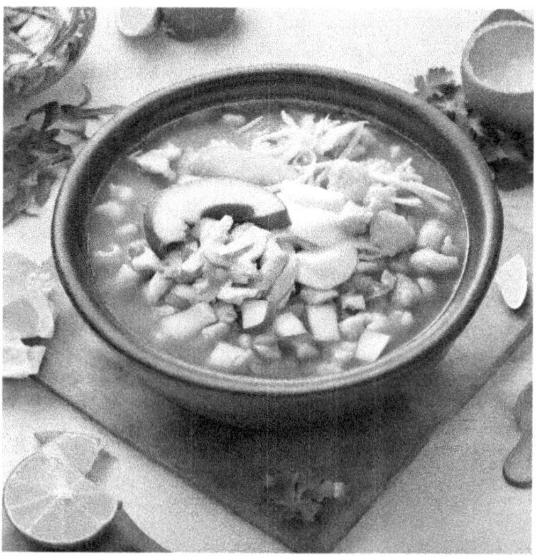

2. Indian Dal Soup

Ingredients:

- 1 cup red lentils, rinsed
- 4 cups vegetable broth
- 1 onion, diced
- 2 cloves garlic, minced
- 1 tablespoon grated ginger
- 1 teaspoon turmeric
- 1 teaspoon cumin
- 1/2 teaspoon chili powder
- Salt to taste
- 2 tablespoons tomato paste
- 1 can (13.5 oz) coconut milk
- Juice of 1 lemon
- Fresh cilantro for garnish

Instructions:

1. In a large pot, combine lentils, vegetable broth, onion, garlic, ginger, turmeric, cumin, chili powder, and salt.
2. Bring to a boil, then reduce heat and simmer until lentils are soft, about 20 minutes.
3. Stir in tomato paste and coconut milk. Continue to simmer for another 10 minutes.
4. Add lemon juice and adjust seasoning as needed.
5. Serve garnished with fresh cilantro.

Nutrition Info per Serving (serves 6):

- Calories: 240
- Protein: 9g
- Carbohydrates: 28g
- Fat: 11g
- Sodium: 300mg
- Fiber: 6g

Cooking Time: 40 minutes

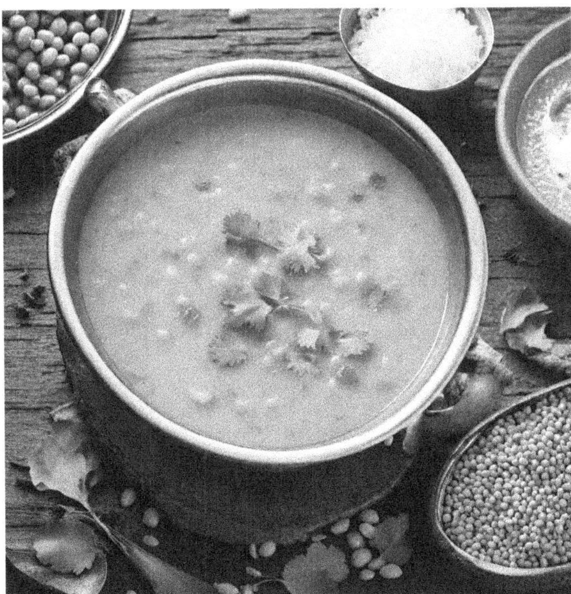

3. Chinese Hot and Sour Soup

Ingredients:

- 4 cups chicken or vegetable broth
- 1/4 cup soy sauce
- 1 tablespoon rice vinegar
- 1 teaspoon ground ginger
- 1 tablespoon cornstarch mixed with 2 tablespoons water
- 1 egg, lightly beaten
- 1/2 cup mushrooms, thinly sliced
- 1/2 cup tofu, cut into small cubes
- 1 bamboo shoot, thinly sliced (optional)
- 1 teaspoon sesame oil
- Salt and pepper to taste
- Green onions and cilantro for garnish

Instructions:

1. In a large pot, bring broth, soy sauce, rice vinegar, and ginger to a simmer.
2. Stir in the cornstarch mixture until the soup thickens slightly.
3. Slowly pour in the beaten egg while stirring the soup to create egg ribbons.
4. Add mushrooms, tofu, and bamboo shoots. Simmer for 5 minutes.
5. Stir in sesame oil, and season with salt and pepper.
6. Serve garnished with green onions and cilantro.

Nutrition Info per Serving (serves 4):

- Calories: 100
- Protein: 7g
- Carbohydrates: 8g
- Fat: 4g
- Sodium: 1100mg
- Fiber: 1g

Cooking Time: 25 minutes

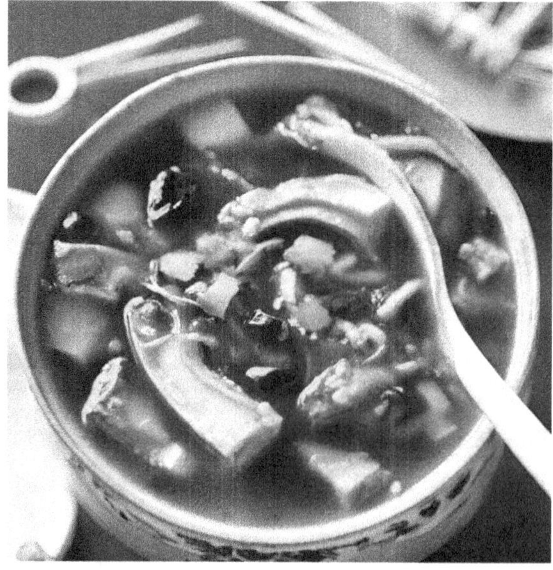

4. French Onion Soup

Ingredients:

- 3 tablespoons butter
- 4 large onions, thinly sliced
- 1 teaspoon sugar
- 1 tablespoon all-purpose flour
- 6 cups beef broth
- 1/2 cup dry white wine
- Salt and pepper to taste
- 4 slices of crusty bread
- 1 cup grated Gruyère cheese

Instructions:

1. In a large pot, melt butter over medium heat. Add onions and sugar, cooking until onions are caramelized, about 30 minutes.
2. Sprinkle flour over onions and stir. Add beef broth and wine. Season with salt and pepper.
3. Bring to a boil, then reduce heat and simmer for 30 minutes.
4. Preheat the broiler. Place bread slices on a baking sheet and broil until toasted. Remove from oven.
5. Ladle soup into oven-safe bowls. Place a slice of toast on top of each, and sprinkle with Gruyère cheese.
6. Broil until cheese is bubbly and golden.
7. Serve immediately.

Nutrition Info per Serving (serves 4):

- Calories: 350
- Protein: 18g
- Carbohydrates: 34g
- Fat: 16g
- Sodium: 900mg
- Fiber: 3g

Cooking Time: 1 hour 10 minutes

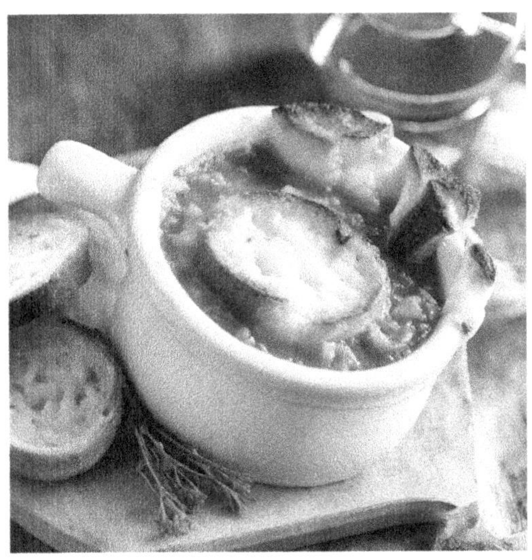

5. Moroccan Harira

Ingredients:

- 2 tablespoons olive oil
- 1 onion, chopped
- 2 celery stalks, chopped
- 2 teaspoons ground cinnamon
- 2 teaspoons ground turmeric
- 1 teaspoon ground ginger
- 1 can (14.5 oz) diced tomatoes
- 1 cup lentils, rinsed
- 6 cups vegetable broth
- 1/2 cup cilantro, chopped
- 1/2 cup parsley, chopped
- 1 can (15 oz) chickpeas, drained and rinsed
- Juice of 1 lemon
- Salt and pepper to taste

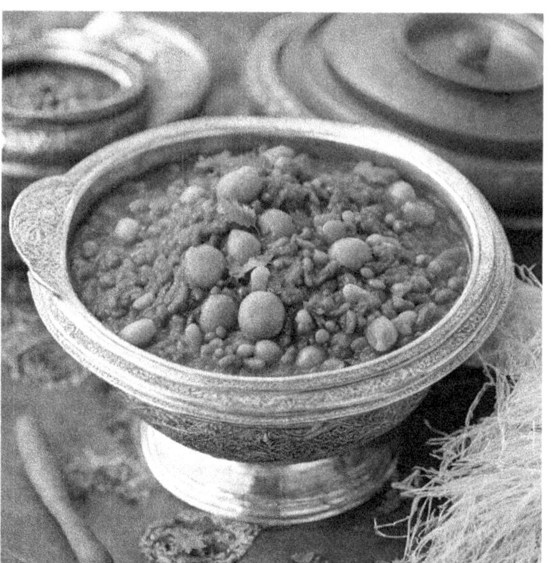

Instructions:

1. In a large pot, heat olive oil over medium heat. Add onion and celery, cooking until softened.
2. Stir in cinnamon, turmeric, and ginger, cooking for another minute.
3. Add diced tomatoes, lentils, and vegetable broth. Bring to a boil, then reduce heat and simmer until lentils are tender, about 30 minutes.
4. Add cilantro, parsley, chickpeas, and lemon juice. Season with salt and pepper.
5. Simmer for an additional 10 minutes.
6. Serve hot.

Nutrition Info per Serving (serves 6):

- Calories: 220
- Protein: 12g
- Carbohydrates: 35g
- Fat: 5g
- Sodium: 800mg
- Fiber: 10g

Cooking Time: 50 minutes

6. Sweet Potato Coconut Soup

Ingredients:

- 2 tablespoons olive oil
- 1 onion, chopped
- 2 cloves garlic, minced
- 2 pounds sweet potatoes, peeled and cubed
- 4 cups vegetable broth
- 1 can (14 oz) coconut milk
- 1 teaspoon ground ginger
- Salt and pepper to taste
- Fresh cilantro for garnish

Instructions:

1. Heat olive oil in a large pot over medium heat. Sauté onion and garlic until soft.
2. Add sweet potatoes, vegetable broth, coconut milk, and ginger. Season with salt and pepper.
3. Bring to a boil, then reduce heat and simmer until sweet potatoes are tender, about 20 minutes.
4. Use an immersion blender to purée the soup until smooth.
5. Serve garnished with fresh cilantro.

Nutrition Info per Serving (serves 6):

- Calories: 350
- Protein: 4g
- Carbohydrates: 45g
- Fat: 18g
- Sodium: 630mg
- Fiber: 6g

Cooking Time: 40 minutes

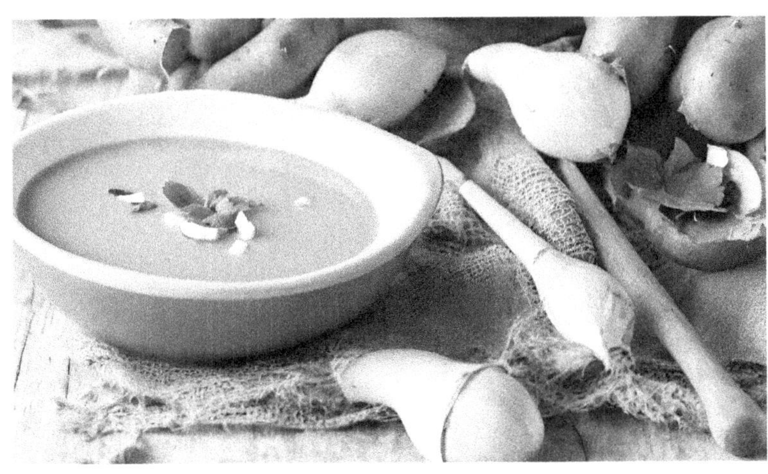

7. Roasted Garlic Cauliflower Soup

Ingredients:

- 1 large head cauliflower, cut into florets
- 3 tablespoons olive oil, divided
- 1 head garlic, top sliced off
- 1 onion, chopped
- 4 cups vegetable broth
- Salt and pepper to taste
- Fresh thyme for garnish

Instructions:

1. Preheat the oven to 400°F (200°C). Toss cauliflower florets with 2 tablespoons olive oil, and spread on a baking sheet. Place garlic head on the same sheet. Roast for 25-30 minutes.
2. Heat the remaining olive oil in a pot over medium heat. Add onion and sauté until soft.
3. Squeeze roasted garlic out of its skin and add to the pot along with roasted cauliflower. Add vegetable broth, salt, and pepper.
4. Simmer for 10-15 minutes. Blend until smooth with an immersion blender.
5. Serve garnished with fresh thyme.

Nutrition Info per Serving (serves 4):

- Calories: 180
- Protein: 4g
- Carbohydrates: 20g
- Fat: 10g
- Sodium: 950mg
- Fiber: 5g

Cooking Time: 50 minutes

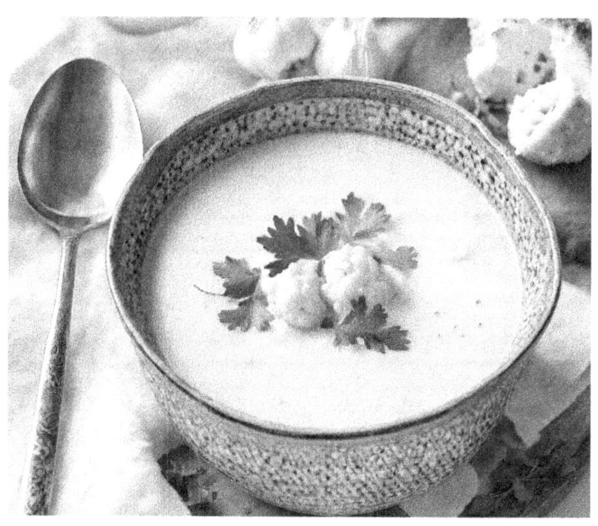

8. Avocado Soup

Ingredients:

- 2 ripe avocados
- 2 cups chicken or vegetable broth, chilled
- 1/2 cup cream or coconut milk
- Juice of 1 lime
- Salt and pepper to taste
- Fresh cilantro for garnish
- Chili flakes for garnish (optional)

Instructions:

1. Blend avocados, broth, cream or coconut milk, and lime juice until smooth. Season with salt and pepper.
2. Chill the soup for at least 1 hour before serving.
3. Serve garnished with fresh cilantro and chili flakes if desired.

Nutrition Info per Serving (serves 4):

- Calories: 250
- Protein: 3g
- Carbohydrates: 12g
- Fat: 22g
- Sodium: 470mg
- Fiber: 7g

Cooking Time: 1 hour 10 minutes (including chilling)

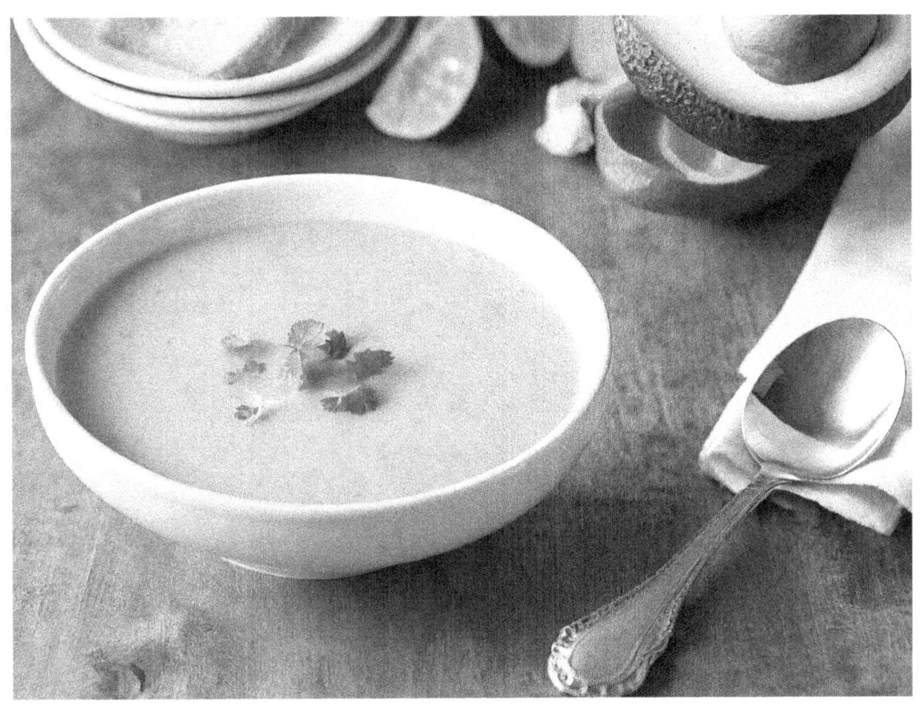

9. Cream of Mushroom Soup

Ingredients:

- 2 tablespoons butter
- 1 onion, chopped
- 2 cloves garlic, minced
- 1 pound mushrooms, sliced
- 4 cups vegetable broth
- 1 cup heavy cream
- Salt and pepper to taste
- Fresh parsley for garnish

Instructions:

1. Melt butter in a large pot over medium heat. Add onion and garlic, sautéing until soft.
2. Add mushrooms and cook until they have released their moisture and browned.
3. Add vegetable broth and bring to a simmer. Cook for 15 minutes.
4. Stir in heavy cream, and blend the soup until smooth. Season with salt and pepper.
5. Serve garnished with fresh parsley.

Nutrition Info per Serving (serves 4):

- Calories: 300
- Protein: 5g
- Carbohydrates: 15g
- Fat: 25g
- Sodium: 950mg
- Fiber: 2g

Cooking Time: 40 minutes

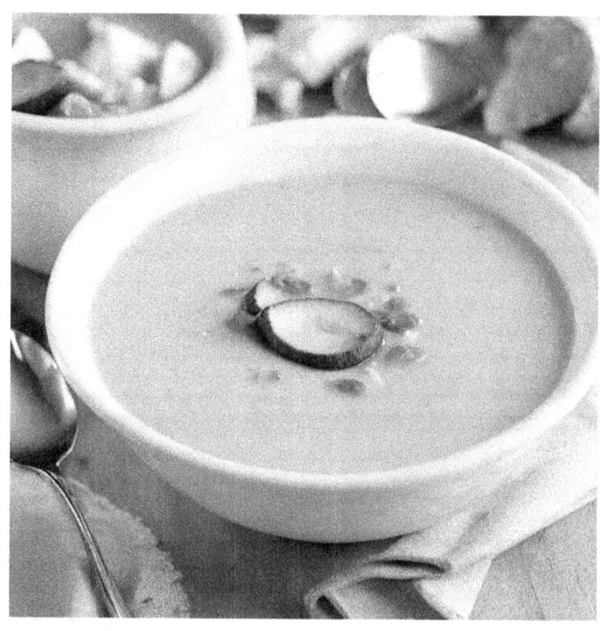

10. West African Peanut Stew

Ingredients:

- 2 tablespoons olive oil
- 1 onion, chopped
- 2 cloves garlic, minced
- 1 sweet potato, peeled and cubed
- 1 bell pepper, chopped
- 1 can (14 oz) diced tomatoes
- 4 cups vegetable broth
- 1/2 cup peanut butter
- 1 teaspoon cayenne pepper (adjust to taste)
- Salt to taste
- 2 cups chopped kale or spinach
- Fresh cilantro for garnish

Instructions:

1. Heat olive oil in a large pot over medium heat. Sauté onion, garlic, sweet potato, and bell pepper until softened.
2. Stir in diced tomatoes, vegetable broth, peanut butter, and cayenne pepper. Season with salt.
3. Bring to a boil, then reduce heat and simmer until sweet potatoes are tender, about 20 minutes.
4. Stir in kale or spinach and cook until wilted.
5. Serve garnished with fresh cilantro.

Nutrition Info per Serving (serves 6):

- Calories: 280
- Protein: 9g
- Carbohydrates: 25g
- Fat: 18g
- Sodium: 630mg
- Fiber: 5g

Cooking Time: 45 minutes

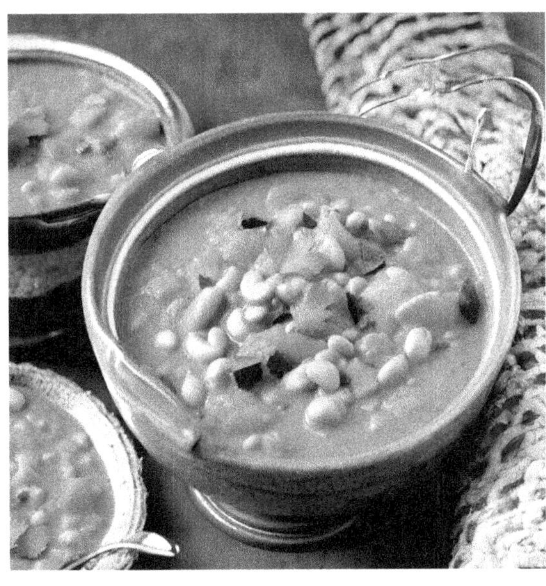

11. Spanish Chickpea and Spinach Stew

Ingredients:

- 2 tablespoons olive oil
- 1 onion, diced
- 3 cloves garlic, minced
- 1 teaspoon smoked paprika
- 1/2 teaspoon cumin
- 2 cans (15 oz each) chickpeas, drained and rinsed
- 1 can (14.5 oz) diced tomatoes
- 4 cups vegetable broth
- 6 cups fresh spinach
- Salt and pepper to taste
- 2 tablespoons red wine vinegar

Instructions:

1. Heat olive oil in a large pot over medium heat. Add onion and garlic, cooking until softened.
2. Stir in smoked paprika and cumin, cooking for another minute.
3. Add chickpeas, diced tomatoes, and vegetable broth. Season with salt and pepper. Bring to a boil, then reduce heat and simmer for 20 minutes.
4. Stir in spinach and cook until wilted, about 3 minutes.
5. Stir in red wine vinegar and adjust seasoning as needed.
6. Serve hot.

Nutrition Info per Serving (serves 6):

- Calories: 230
- Protein: 9g
- Carbohydrates: 35g
- Fat: 6g
- Sodium: 700mg
- Fiber: 9g

Cooking Time: 35 minutes

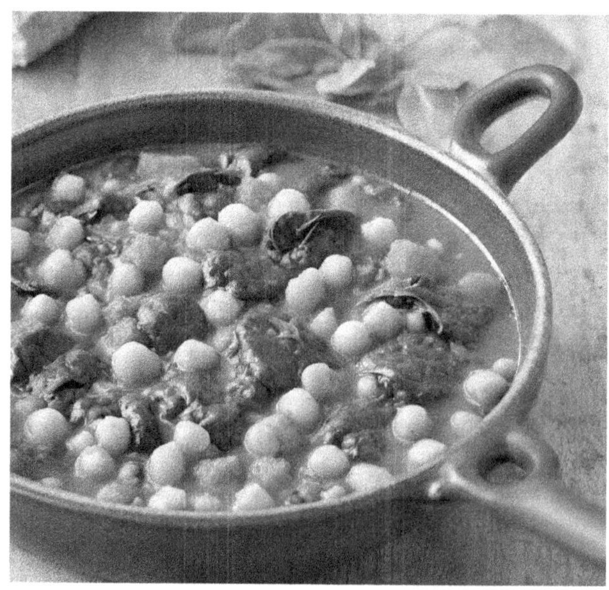

12. Cuban Black Bean Stew

Ingredients:

- 2 tablespoons olive oil
- 1 onion, chopped
- 1 bell pepper, chopped
- 3 cloves garlic, minced
- 2 cans (15 oz each) black beans, undrained
- 2 cups vegetable broth
- 1 teaspoon cumin
- 1/2 teaspoon oregano
- Salt and pepper to taste
- Juice of 1 lime
- Fresh cilantro for garnish

Instructions:

1. Heat olive oil in a pot over medium heat. Add onion, bell pepper, and garlic, sautéing until soft.
2. Add black beans (with their liquid), vegetable broth, cumin, and oregano. Season with salt and pepper.
3. Bring to a boil, then reduce heat and simmer for 30 minutes, partially covered. For a thicker stew, mash some of the beans with a spoon.
4. Stir in lime juice before serving.
5. Garnish with fresh cilantro.

Nutrition Info per Serving (serves 6):

- Calories: 220
- Protein: 11g
- Carbohydrates: 35g
- Fat: 5g
- Sodium: 470mg
- Fiber: 10g

Cooking Time: 45 minutes

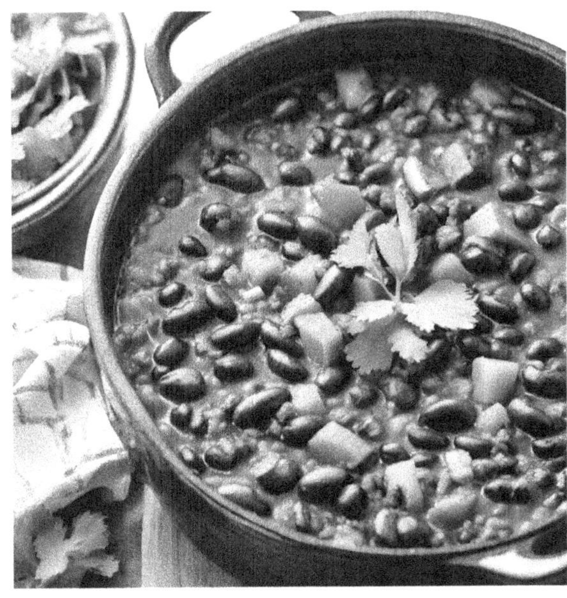

13. Ethiopian Lentil Stew (Misir Wot)

Ingredients:

- 2 tablespoons olive oil
- 1 onion, finely chopped
- 3 cloves garlic, minced
- 1 tablespoon berbere spice mix
- 1 cup red lentils, rinsed
- 2 cups vegetable broth
- 1 can (14.5 oz) diced tomatoes
- Salt to taste
- Fresh cilantro for garnish

Instructions:

1. Heat olive oil in a pot over medium heat. Add onion and garlic, cooking until soft.
2. Stir in berbere spice mix, cooking for another minute.
3. Add lentils, vegetable broth, and diced tomatoes. Season with salt.
4. Bring to a boil, then reduce heat and simmer until lentils are soft, about 20 minutes.
5. Garnish with fresh cilantro before serving.

Nutrition Info per Serving (serves 4):

- Calories: 270
- Protein: 14g
- Carbohydrates: 40g
- Fat: 7g
- Sodium: 300mg
- Fiber: 18g

Cooking Time: 35 minutes

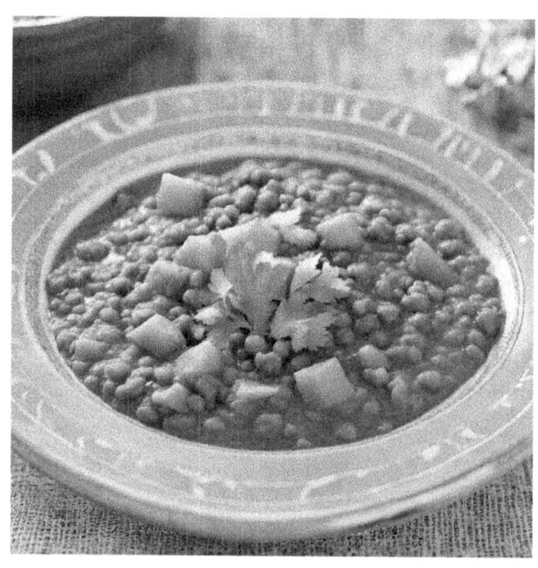

14. Italian Bean Stew

Ingredients:

- 2 tablespoons olive oil
- 1 onion, chopped
- 2 carrots, diced
- 2 stalks celery, diced
- 3 cloves garlic, minced
- 2 cans (15 oz each) cannellini beans, rinsed and drained
- 4 cups vegetable broth
- 1 teaspoon dried thyme
- Salt and pepper to taste
- Fresh parsley, chopped for garnish
- Grated Parmesan cheese for serving

Instructions:

1. Heat olive oil in a pot over medium heat. Add onion, carrots, celery, and garlic, cooking until vegetables are soft.
2. Add cannellini beans, vegetable broth, and thyme. Season with salt and pepper.
3. Bring to a boil, then reduce heat and simmer for 30 minutes.
4. Serve garnished with fresh parsley and grated Parmesan cheese.

Nutrition Info per Serving (serves 6):

- Calories: 200
- Protein: 10g
- Carbohydrates: 30g
- Fat: 5g
- Sodium: 800mg
- Fiber: 8g

Cooking Time: 45 minutes

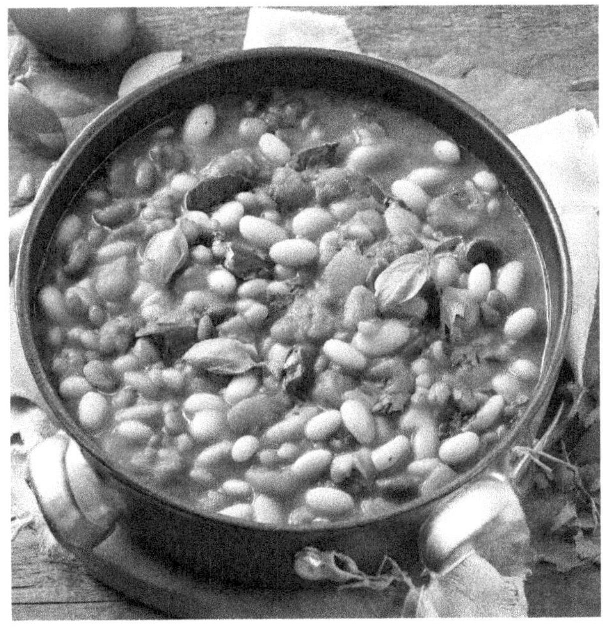

15. Irish Beef Stew

Ingredients:
- 2 tablespoons olive oil
- 1.5 pounds beef stew meat, cut into chunks
- 3 tablespoons flour
- 3 carrots, peeled and sliced
- 3 potatoes, peeled and cubed
- 1 onion, chopped
- 4 cups beef broth
- 1 cup stout beer (optional)
- 2 teaspoons thyme
- Salt and pepper to taste
- Fresh parsley, chopped for garnish

Instructions:
1. Toss beef chunks with flour, salt, and pepper. Heat olive oil in a large pot over medium-high heat. Add beef and brown on all sides.
2. Add carrots, potatoes, onion, beef broth, stout beer (if using), and thyme. Season with additional salt and pepper.
3. Bring to a boil, then reduce heat and simmer, covered, until beef is tender, about 2 hours.
4. Garnish with fresh parsley before serving.

Nutrition Info per Serving (serves 6):
- Calories: 420
- Protein: 35g
- Carbohydrates: 35g
- Fat: 15g
- Sodium: 650mg
- Fiber: 5g

Cooking Time: 2 hours 30 minutes

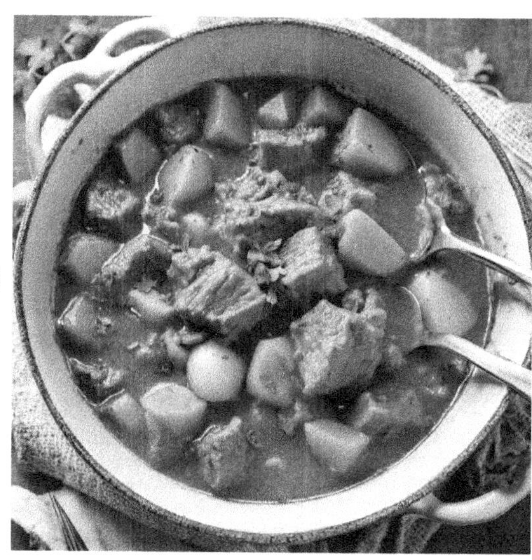

16. Hungarian Mushroom Soup

Ingredients:

- 2 tablespoons butter
- 1 large onion, chopped
- 1 pound mushrooms, sliced
- 2 teaspoons dried dill weed
- 1 tablespoon paprika
- 1 tablespoon soy sauce
- 2 cups vegetable broth
- 1 cup milk
- 3 tablespoons all-purpose flour
- 1/2 cup sour cream
- Salt and pepper to taste
- Fresh parsley, chopped for garnish

Instructions:

1. Melt butter in a large pot over medium heat. Add onion, cooking until soft.
2. Add mushrooms, dill, paprika, and soy sauce. Cook until mushrooms are soft.
3. Stir in vegetable broth and bring to a simmer.
4. In a small bowl, whisk together milk and flour until smooth. Gradually stir into the soup.
5. Simmer for 15 minutes, stirring frequently. Remove from heat.
6. Stir in sour cream and season with salt and pepper.
7. Serve garnished with fresh parsley.

Nutrition Info per Serving (serves 6):

- Calories: 150
- Protein: 5g
- Carbohydrates: 13g
- Fat: 9g
- Sodium: 570mg
- Fiber: 2g

Cooking Time: 35 minutes

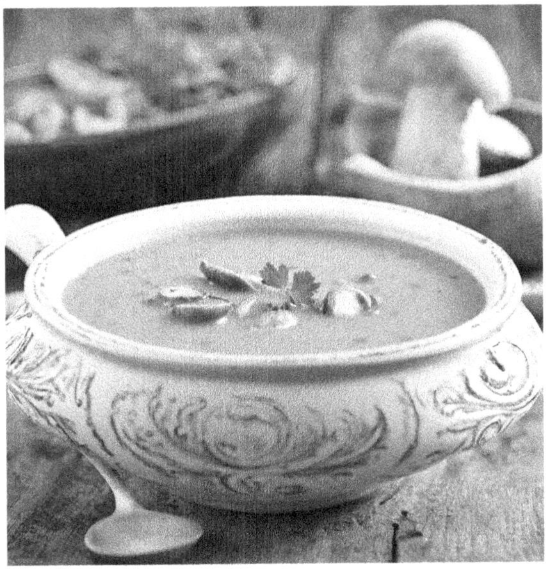

17. Norwegian Fish Soup (Fiskesuppe)

Ingredients:

- 2 tablespoons butter
- 1 onion, finely chopped
- 2 carrots, sliced
- 2 cups fish stock
- 1 cup water
- 1 pound mixed fish fillets (cod, salmon, haddock), cut into pieces
- 1/2 cup heavy cream
- Salt and white pepper to taste
- Fresh dill, chopped for garnish

Instructions:

1. Melt butter in a large pot over medium heat. Add onion and carrots, cooking until soft.
2. Add fish stock and water, bringing to a simmer.
3. Add fish pieces and simmer gently until cooked through, about 10 minutes.
4. Stir in heavy cream and season with salt and white pepper.
5. Serve garnished with fresh dill.

Nutrition Info per Serving (serves 4):

- Calories: 300
- Protein: 25g
- Carbohydrates: 6g
- Fat: 20g
- Sodium: 590mg
- Fiber: 1g

Cooking Time: 25 minutes

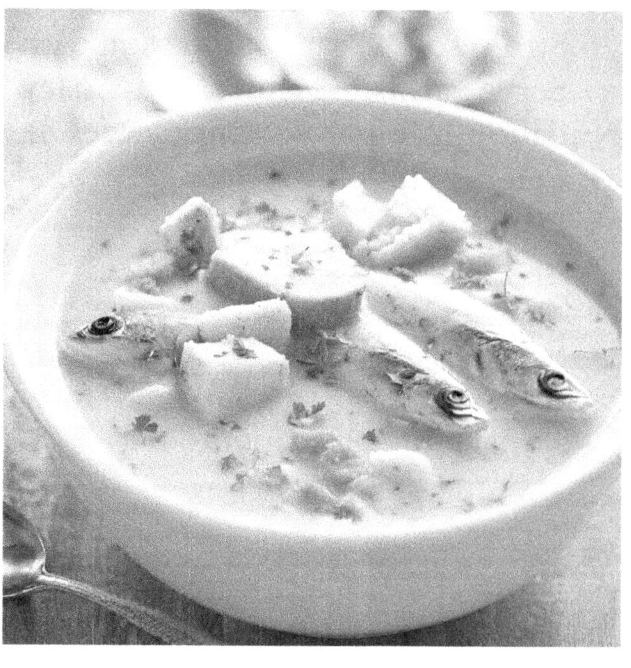

18. Chinese Wonton Soup

Ingredients for Wontons:

- 1/2 pound ground pork
- 1/4 cup shrimp, chopped
- 1 teaspoon soy sauce
- 1 teaspoon sesame oil
- 1/2 teaspoon ginger, minced
- 1 green onion, finely chopped
- Wonton wrappers

Ingredients for Soup:

- 4 cups chicken broth
- 2 cups water
- 1 tablespoon soy sauce
- 1 tablespoon sesame oil
- 1/2 cup mushrooms, sliced
- Green onions, sliced for garnish

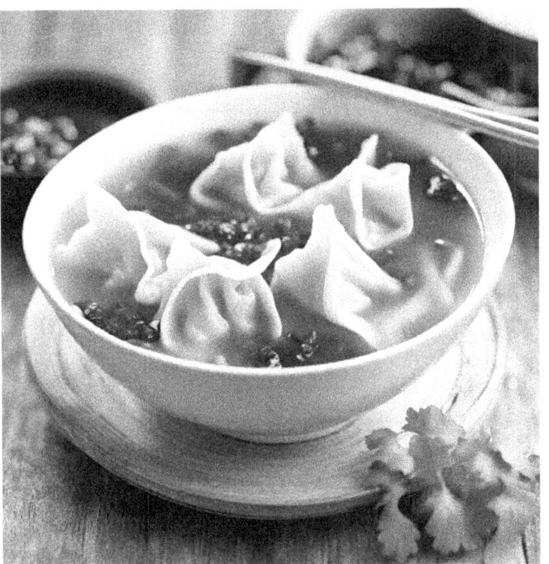

Instructions:

1. Mix ground pork, shrimp, soy sauce, sesame oil, ginger, and green onion in a bowl.
2. Place a teaspoon of filling in the center of each wonton wrapper. Moisten edges with water, fold to enclose the filling, and press to seal.
3. Bring chicken broth and water to a boil in a large pot. Add soy sauce and sesame oil.
4. Add wontons and mushrooms to the pot. Simmer until wontons are cooked through, about 5 minutes.
5. Serve garnished with green onions.

Nutrition Info per Serving (serves 4):

- Calories: 280
- Protein: 20g
- Carbohydrates: 22g
- Fat: 12g
- Sodium: 1100mg
- Fiber: 1g

Cooking Time: 45 minutes

19. Korean Seaweed Soup (Miyeok Guk)

Ingredients:

- 1/2 cup dried seaweed (miyeok), soaked and cut into pieces
- 1 tablespoon sesame oil
- 1/2 pound beef, thinly sliced
- 4 cups water
- 2 cloves garlic, minced
- 2 tablespoons soy sauce
- Salt to taste
- Sesame seeds for garnish

Instructions:

1. Heat sesame oil in a pot over medium heat. Add beef and garlic, cooking until beef is browned.
2. Add soaked seaweed and water. Bring to a boil, then reduce heat and simmer for 20 minutes.
3. Stir in soy sauce and season with salt.
4. Serve garnished with sesame seeds.

Nutrition Info per Serving (serves 4):

- Calories: 150
- Protein: 15g
- Carbohydrates: 3g
- Fat: 8g
- Sodium: 870mg
- Fiber: 1g

Cooking Time: 30 minutes

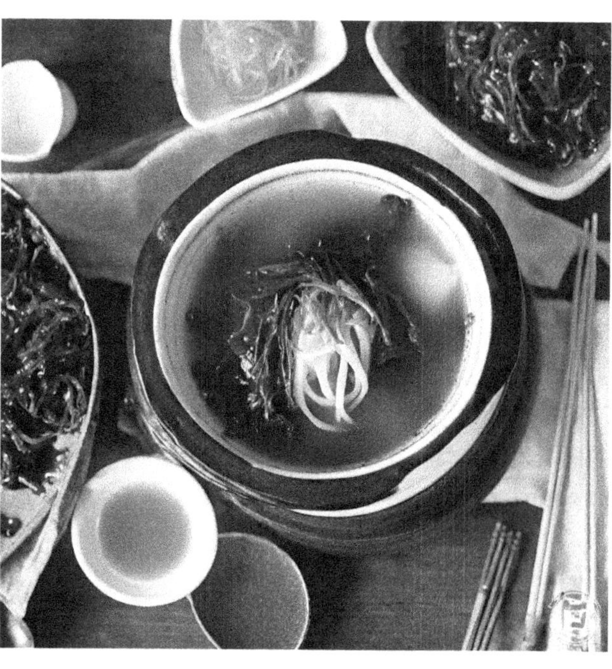

20. Polish Mushroom Barley Soup

Ingredients:

- 1 cup pearl barley, rinsed
- 2 tablespoons olive oil
- 1 onion, chopped
- 2 carrots, diced
- 2 celery stalks, diced
- 1 pound mushrooms, sliced
- 6 cups vegetable broth
- Salt and pepper to taste
- Fresh parsley, chopped for garnish

Instructions:

1. In a large pot, cook barley in boiling water for 30 minutes. Drain and set aside.
2. Heat olive oil in the same pot. Add onion, carrots, and celery, cooking until soft.
3. Add mushrooms and cook until browned.
4. Add cooked barley and vegetable broth. Season with salt and pepper.
5. Bring to a boil, then reduce heat and simmer for 20 minutes.
6. Serve garnished with fresh parsley.

Nutrition Info per Serving (serves 6):

- Calories: 220
- Protein: 7g
- Carbohydrates: 42g
- Fat: 4g
- Sodium: 950mg
- Fiber: 9g

Cooking Time: 1 hour 10 minutes

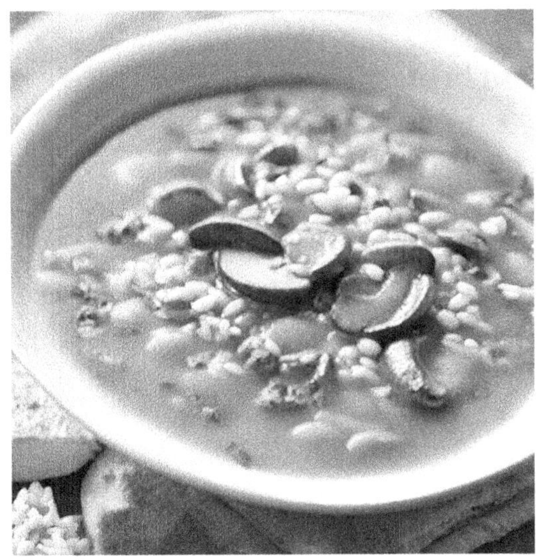

21. Cheddar and Ale Soup

Ingredients:

- 2 tablespoons butter
- 1 onion, chopped
- 2 carrots, diced
- 2 celery stalks, diced
- 2 cloves garlic, minced
- 1/4 cup all-purpose flour
- 1 cup ale or beer
- 4 cups chicken or vegetable broth
- 2 cups shredded sharp cheddar cheese
- 1 cup heavy cream
- Salt and pepper to taste
- Fresh thyme for garnish

Instructions:

1. Melt butter in a large pot over medium heat. Add onion, carrots, celery, and garlic, cooking until softened.
2. Stir in flour to create a roux. Gradually whisk in ale, then broth, until smooth.
3. Bring to a simmer, cooking until vegetables are tender.
4. Reduce heat to low. Stir in cheddar cheese until melted. Stir in heavy cream. Season with salt and pepper.
5. Serve garnished with fresh thyme.

Nutrition Info per Serving (serves 6):

- Calories: 400
- Protein: 15g
- Carbohydrates: 15g
- Fat: 30g
- Sodium: 850mg
- Fiber: 2g

Cooking Time: 40 minutes

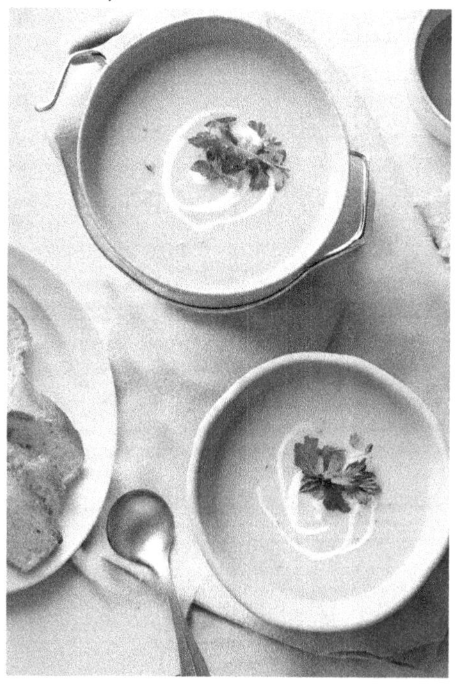

SMOOTHIES

1. Strawberry Banana Bliss
Ingredients:
- 1 cup strawberries, fresh or frozen
- 1 ripe banana
- 1/2 cup Greek yogurt
- 1/2 cup orange juice
- 1 tablespoon honey (optional)

Instructions:
1. Combine strawberries, banana, Greek yogurt, orange juice, and honey (if using) in a blender.
2. Blend until smooth.
3. Serve immediately.

Nutrition Info per Serving (serves 2):
- Calories: 150
- Protein: 5g
- Carbohydrates: 34g
- Fat: 0.5g
- Sodium: 20mg
- Fiber: 3g

Cooking Time: 5 minutes

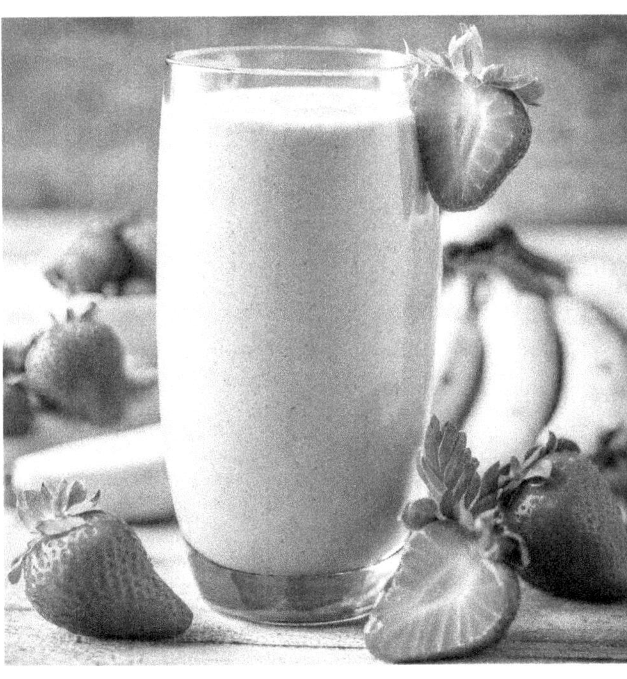

2. Blueberry Muffin Smoothie

Ingredients:
- 1 cup blueberries, fresh or frozen
- 1 banana
- 1/2 cup oats
- 1 cup almond milk
- 1 tablespoon maple syrup
- 1/2 teaspoon vanilla extract
- Dash of cinnamon

Instructions:
1. Combine blueberries, banana, oats, almond milk, maple syrup, vanilla extract, and cinnamon in a blender.
2. Blend until smooth.
3. Serve immediately.

Nutrition Info per Serving (serves 2):
- Calories: 220 Protein: 4g Carbohydrates: 46g Fat: 3g
- Sodium: 80mg Fiber: 6g

Cooking Time: 5 minutes

3. Kale Pineapple Hydrator

Ingredients:
- 2 cups kale, stems removed
- 1 cup pineapple, chopped
- 1 banana
- 1/2 cucumber, sliced
- 1 cup coconut water
- Juice of 1/2 lime

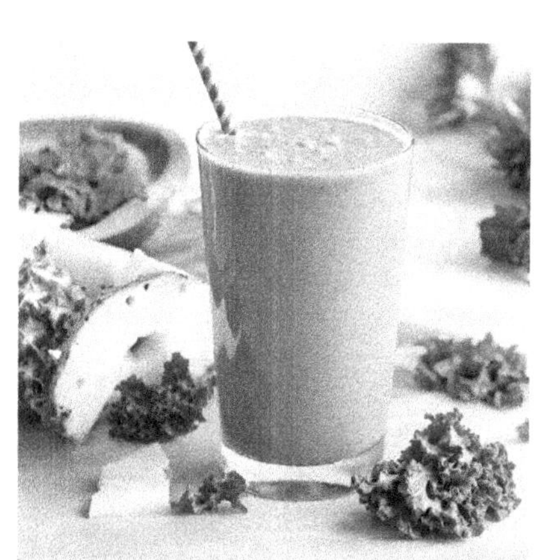

Instructions:
1. Combine kale, pineapple, banana, cucumber, coconut water, and lime juice in a blender.
2. Blend until smooth.
3. Serve immediately.

Nutrition Info per Serving (serves 2):
- Calories: 140 Protein: 3g Carbohydrates: 34g
- Fat: 0.5g
- Sodium: 60mg
- Fiber: 5g

Cooking Time: 5 minutes

4. Spinach Avocado Bliss

Ingredients:

- 2 cups spinach
- 1/2 avocado
- 1 banana
- 1 cup almond milk
- 1 tablespoon chia seeds
- 1 tablespoon honey (optional)

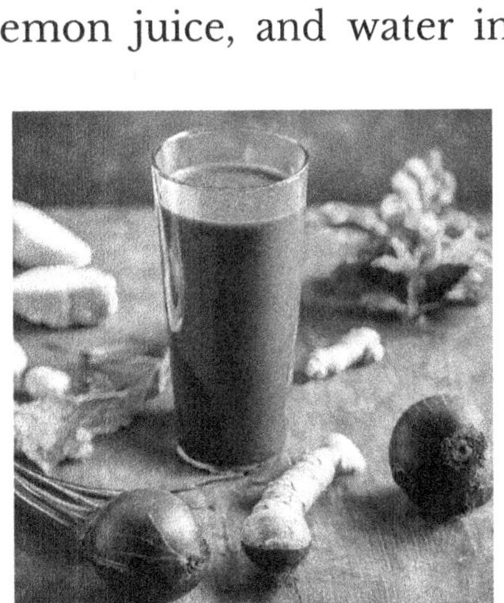

Instructions:

1. Combine spinach, avocado, banana, almond milk, chia seeds, and honey (if using) in a blender.
2. Blend until smooth.
3. Serve immediately.

Nutrition Info per Serving (serves 2):

- Calories: 200 Protein: 4g Carbohydrates: 30g Fat: 9g
- Sodium: 90mg Fiber: 7g

Cooking Time: 5 minutes

5. Beetroot Ginger Detox

Ingredients:

- 1 medium beetroot, peeled and chopped
- 1 apple, cored and chopped
- 1/2 inch piece of ginger, peeled
- 1/2 lemon, juiced
- 1 cup water

Instructions:

1. Combine beetroot, apple, ginger, lemon juice, and water in a blender.
2. Blend until smooth.
3. Serve immediately.

Nutrition Info per Serving (serves 2):

- Calories: 90
- Protein: 2g
- Carbohydrates: 22g
- Fat: 0.2g
- Sodium: 60mg
- Fiber: 5g

Cooking Time: 5 minutes

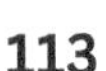

6. Carrot Cake Smoothie

Ingredients:
- 1 cup carrots, chopped
- 1 banana
- 1/4 cup walnuts
- 1 cup almond milk
- 1/2 teaspoon cinnamon
- 1/4 teaspoon nutmeg
- 1 tablespoon maple syrup

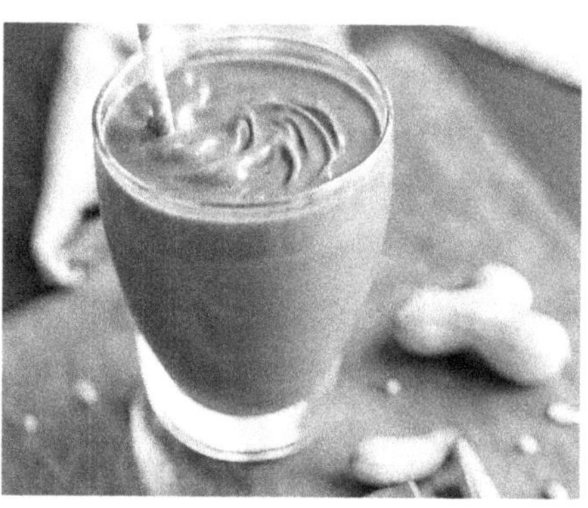

Instructions:
1. Combine carrots, banana, walnuts, almond milk, cinnamon, nutmeg, and maple syrup in a blender.
2. Blend until smooth.
3. Serve immediately.

Nutrition Info per Serving (serves 2):
- Calories: 220 Protein: 4g Carbohydrates: 30g Fat: 11g
- Sodium: 80mg Fiber: 4g

Cooking Time: 5 minutes

7. Chocolate Peanut Butter Protein

Ingredients:
- 1 banana, frozen
- 2 tablespoons peanut butter
- 1 tablespoon cocoa powder
- 1 cup almond milk
- 1 scoop protein powder (chocolate or vanilla)
- Ice cubes (optional)

Instructions:
1. Combine the banana, peanut butter, cocoa powder, almond milk, protein powder, and ice cubes (if using) in a blender.
2. Blend until smooth and creamy.
3. Serve immediately.

Nutrition Info per Serving (serves 2):
- Calories: 280 Protein: 15g Carbohydrates: 30g Fat: 14g
- Sodium: 180mg
- Fiber: 5g

Cooking Time: 5 minutes

8. Vanilla Berry Protein Blast

Ingredients:

- 1 cup mixed berries (strawberries, blueberries, raspberries), fresh or frozen
- 1 banana
- 1 cup Greek yogurt
- 1 scoop vanilla protein powder
- 1 teaspoon vanilla extract
- 1 cup almond milk

Instructions:

1. Combine mixed berries, banana, Greek yogurt, protein powder, vanilla extract, and almond milk in a blender.
2. Blend until smooth.
3. Serve immediately.

Nutrition Info per Serving (serves 2):

- Calories: 250 Protein: 20g Carbohydrates: 35g Fat: 2g
- Sodium: 100mg Fiber: 4g

Cooking Time: 5 minutes

9. Acai Berry Antioxidant

Ingredients:

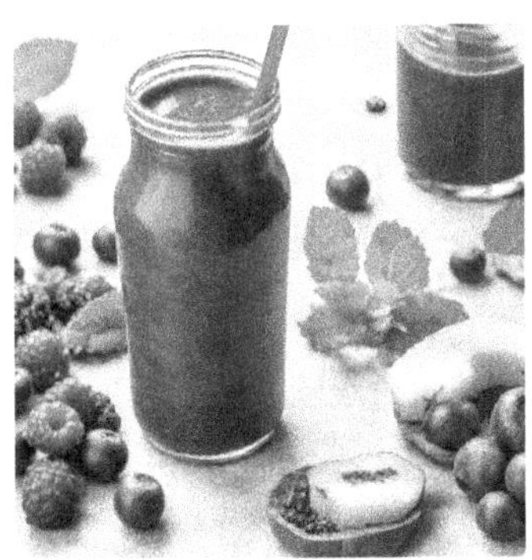

- 1 acai berry smoothie pack, unsweetened
- 1/2 banana
- 1/2 cup mixed berries
- 1 tablespoon flaxseeds
- 1 cup spinach leaves
- 1 cup coconut water

Instructions:

1. Combine the acai smoothie pack, banana, mixed berries, flaxseeds, spinach, and coconut water in a blender.
2. Blend until smooth.
3. Serve immediately.

Nutrition Info per Serving (serves 2):

- Calories: 150 Protein: 2g Carbohydrates: 30g Fat: 3g
- Sodium: 30mg   Fiber: 7g

Cooking Time: 5 minutes

10. Golden Turmeric Healing

Ingredients:

- 1 cup coconut milk
- 1/2 banana
- 1/2 teaspoon turmeric powder
- 1/4 teaspoon ginger powder
- 1 tablespoon honey
- Pinch of black pepper
- Ice cubes (optional)

Instructions:

1. Combine coconut milk, banana, turmeric powder, ginger powder, honey, black pepper, and ice cubes (if using) in a blender.
2. Blend until smooth.
3. Serve immediately.

Nutrition Info per Serving (serves 2):

- Calories: 180 Protein: 2g Carbohydrates: 25g Fat: 9g
- Sodium: 20mg Fiber: 2g

Cooking Time: 5 minutes

11. Watermelon Wonder

Ingredients:

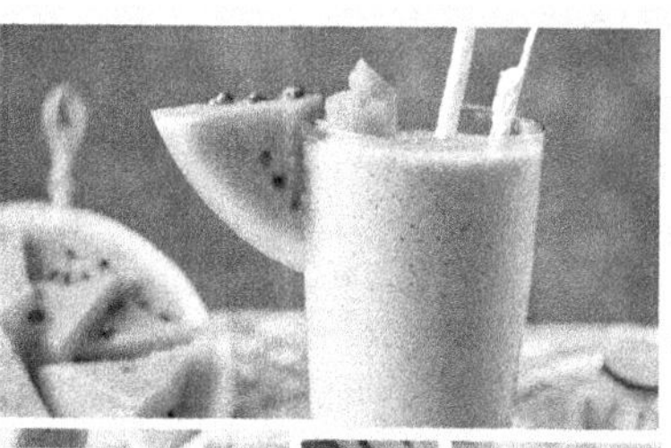

- 2 cups watermelon, cubed
- 1/2 cup strawberries, fresh or frozen
- 1/2 cup Greek yogurt
- Juice of 1 lime
- Mint leaves for garnish

Instructions:

1. Combine watermelon, strawberries, Greek yogurt, and lime juice in a blender.
2. Blend until smooth.
3. Serve garnished with mint leaves.

Nutrition Info per Serving (serves 2):

- Calories: 120 Protein: 7g Carbohydrates: 23g Fat: 0.5g
- Sodium: 35mg Fiber: 2g

Cooking Time: 5 minutes

12. Coconut Cucumber Splash

Ingredients:

- 1 cup cucumber, chopped
- 1/2 cup coconut water
- 1/2 cup pineapple, chopped
- 1/2 banana
- Juice of 1/2 lime
- Fresh mint leaves

Instructions:

1. Combine cucumber, coconut water, pineapple, banana, lime juice, and mint leaves in a blender.
2. Blend until smooth.
3. Serve immediately.

Nutrition Info per Serving (serves 2):

- Calories: 100 Protein: 1g Carbohydrates: 25g Fat: 0.5g
- Sodium: 30mg Fiber: 3g

Cooking Time: 5 minutes

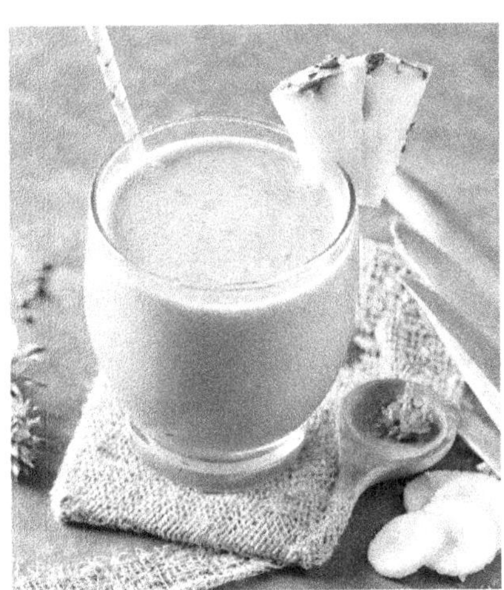

13. Sage Pineapple Digestive

Ingredients:

- 1 cup pineapple, chopped
- 1/2 banana
- 1 tablespoon fresh sage leaves
- 1 cup spinach leaves
- 1 cup coconut water
- 1 tablespoon chia seeds

Instructions:

1. Combine all ingredients in a blender.
2. Blend until smooth and creamy.
3. Serve immediately.

Nutrition Info per Serving (serves 2):

- Calories: 140
- Protein: 2g
- Carbohydrates: 30g
- Fat: 2g
- Sodium: 60mg
- Fiber: 5g

Cooking Time: 5 minutes

14. Rosewater Raspberry

Ingredients:

- 1 cup raspberries, fresh or frozen
- 1 banana
- 1 cup almond milk
- 1 teaspoon rosewater
- 1 tablespoon honey (optional)

Instructions:

1. Combine raspberries, banana, almond milk, rosewater, and honey (if using) in a blender.
2. Blend until smooth.
3. Serve immediately.

Nutrition Info per Serving (serves 2):

- Calories: 150 Protein: 2g Carbohydrates: 35g Fat: 2g
- Sodium: 80mg Fiber: 7g

Cooking Time: 5 minutes

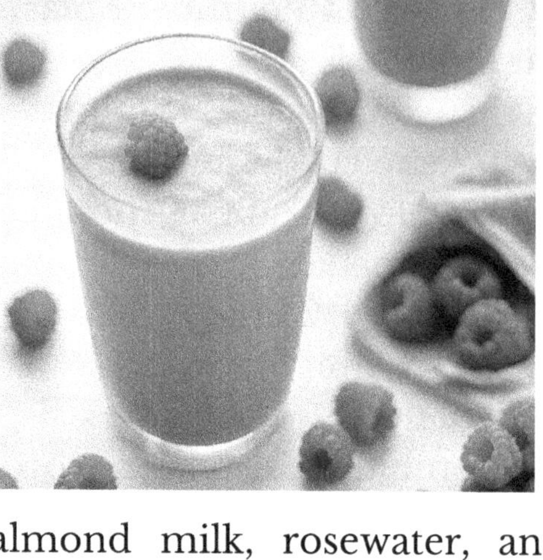

15. Lychee Rose Smoothie

Ingredients:

- 1 cup lychees, peeled and pitted
- 1/2 cup raspberries
- 1/2 banana
- 1 cup coconut milk
- 1 teaspoon rosewater

Instructions:

1. Combine lychees, raspberries, banana, coconut milk, and rosewater in a blender.
2. Blend until smooth.
3. Serve immediately.

Nutrition Info per Serving (serves 2):

- Calories: 200 Protein: 2g Carbohydrates: 30g Fat: 9g
- Sodium: 15mg Fiber: 3g

Cooking Time: 5 minutes

16. Pomegranate Berry Blast

Ingredients:

- 1/2 cup pomegranate seeds
- 1/2 cup mixed berries, fresh or frozen
- 1 banana
- 1 cup spinach leaves
- 1 cup almond milk
- 1 tablespoon flaxseed meal

Instructions:

1. Combine pomegranate seeds, mixed berries, banana, spinach, almond milk, and flaxseed meal in a blender.
2. Blend until smooth.
3. Serve immediately.

Nutrition Info per Serving (serves 2):

- Calories: 180 Protein: 3g Carbohydrates: 35g Fat: 4g
- Sodium: 90mg Fiber: 6g

Cooking Time: 5 minutes

17. Peanut Butter Cup Smoothie

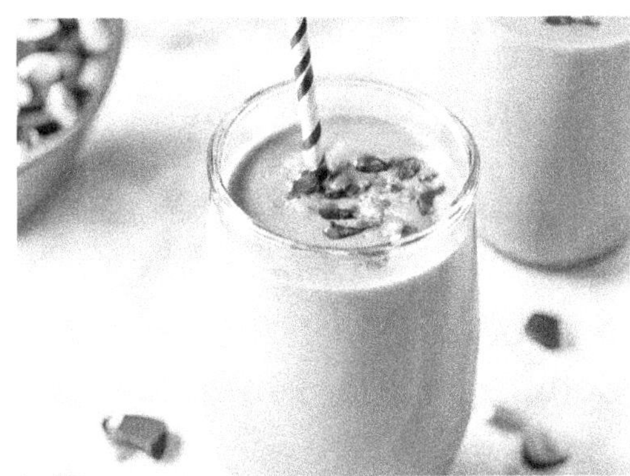

Ingredients:

- 1 banana, frozen
- 2 tablespoons peanut butter
- 1 tablespoon cocoa powder
- 1 cup almond milk
- 1 tablespoon honey (optional)

Instructions:

1. Combine the banana, peanut butter, cocoa powder, almond milk, and honey (if using) in a blender.
2. Blend until smooth and creamy.
3. Serve immediately.

Nutrition Info per Serving (serves 2):

- Calories: 280
- Protein: 8g
- Carbohydrates: 34g
- Fat: 14g
- Sodium: 180mg
- Fiber: 5g

Cooking Time: 5 minutes

Flaxseed Omega Booster Smoothie
Ingredients:
- 1 banana, frozen
- 1 cup blueberries, fresh or frozen
- 2 tablespoons ground flaxseeds
- 1 cup spinach leaves
- 1 tablespoon chia seeds
- 1 cup almond milk
- 1 teaspoon honey (optional)

Instructions:
1. Place the banana, blueberries, ground flaxseeds, spinach, chia seeds, almond milk, and honey (if using) in a blender.
2. Blend on high until smooth and creamy. If the smoothie is too thick, add a little more almond milk until you reach your desired consistency.
3. Serve immediately, enjoying the rich, omega-3-packed boost to start your day or as a nourishing snack.

Nutrition Info per Serving (serves 2):
- Calories: 220
- Protein: 5g
- Carbohydrates: 35g
- Fat: 8g (with high omega-3 content from flaxseeds and chia seeds)
- Sodium: 80mg
- Fiber: 9g

Cooking Time: 5 minutes

8-WEEK MEAL PLAN.

Week 1

Day 1
- **Breakfast:** Strawberry Banana Bliss Smoothie
- **Lunch:** Turkey and Avocado Wrap with a side of Cucumber Ribbon Salad
- **Dinner:** Grilled Salmon with Steamed Broccoli and Quinoa

Day 2
- **Breakfast:** Overnight Oats with Blueberries and Honey
- **Lunch:** Carrot Ginger Soup with a side of Whole Grain Bread
- **Dinner:** Baked Cod with Roasted Vegetables and Sweet Potato Mash

Day 3
- **Breakfast:** Greek Yogurt Parfait with Granola and Mixed Berries
- **Lunch:** Spinach and Strawberry Salad with Grilled Chicken Strips
- **Dinner:** Vegetable Stir-Fry with Tofu over Brown Rice

Day 4
- **Breakfast:** Avocado Toast on Gluten-Free Bread with a Side of Watermelon
- **Lunch:** Tomato Basil Bisque with a side of Arugula and Peach Salad
- **Dinner:** Lemon Dill Salmon Patties with Asparagus Cream Soup

Day 5
- **Breakfast:** Smoothie Bowl with Spinach, Kiwi, Pineapple, and Coconut Flakes
- **Lunch:** Mediterranean Quinoa Salad with Lemon Dressing
- **Dinner:** Chicken and Dumplings Stew

Day 6
- **Breakfast:** Scrambled Eggs with Spinach and Mushrooms on Soft Whole-Grain Toast
- **Lunch:** Butternut Squash Soup with a side of Roasted Garlic Cauliflower
- **Dinner:** Quinoa Stuffed Bell Peppers

Day 7
- **Breakfast:** Blueberry Muffin Smoothie
- **Lunch:** Greek Lemon Chicken Soup
- **Dinner:** Baked Trout with Almond Crust and Steamed Green Beans

Week 2

Day 8
- **Breakfast:** Chia Pudding with Mango and Coconut Milk
- **Lunch:** Chickpea Salad with Cucumbers, Tomatoes, and Feta Cheese
- **Dinner:** Creamy Polenta with Roasted Vegetables

Day 9
- **Breakfast:** Peachy Keen Smoothie
- **Lunch:** Lentil Soup with a side of Warm Pita Bread
- **Dinner:** Grilled Chicken Breast with Quinoa and Roasted Brussels Sprouts

Day 10
- **Breakfast:** Oatmeal with Sliced Bananas, Almond Butter, and Cinnamon
- **Lunch:** Avocado Chicken Salad served in Lettuce Wraps
- **Dinner:** Baked Sweet Potato topped with Black Beans, Corn, and Salsa

Day 11
- **Breakfast:** Cottage Cheese with Pineapple Chunks
- **Lunch:** Cream of Mushroom Soup with a side of Kale Salad
- **Dinner:** Vegetable Lasagna with a Side of Garlic Roasted Broccoli

Day 12
- **Breakfast:** Kiwi Quencher Smoothie
- **Lunch:** Tuna Salad Stuffed Avocados
- **Dinner:** Moroccan Harira with Whole Grain Bread

Day 13
- **Breakfast:** Soft Scrambled Eggs with Avocado and Salsa on Soft Corn Tortillas
- **Lunch:** Sweet Potato Coconut Soup
- **Dinner:** Lemon Butter Baked Cod with Mashed Cauliflower

Day 14
- **Breakfast:** Pomegranate Berry Blast Smoothie
- **Lunch:** Vegetable Minestrone Soup
- **Dinner:** Roasted Chicken with Sweet Potato and Green Bean Almondine

Week 3

Day 1
- **Breakfast:** Pear and Ginger Smoothie
- **Lunch:** Roasted Beet and Goat Cheese Salad
- **Dinner:** Herb-Roasted Chicken Thighs with Steamed Zucchini

Day 2
- **Breakfast:** Vanilla Almond Porridge with Stewed Apples
- **Lunch:** Cold Noodle Salad with Peanut Sauce and Veggies
- **Dinner:** Baked Tilapia with Lemon Herb Quinoa

Day 3
- **Breakfast:** Pineapple and Spinach Green Smoothie
- **Lunch:** Mediterranean Lentil Salad
- **Dinner:** Vegetarian Chili with Avocado and Cornbread

Day 4
- **Breakfast:** Soft Boiled Eggs with Asparagus Soldiers
- **Lunch:** Butternut Squash and Apple Soup
- **Dinner:** Ginger Soy Salmon with Broccoli Rice

Day 5
- **Breakfast:** Banana and Walnut Yogurt Parfait
- **Lunch:** Quinoa Tabbouleh
- **Dinner:** Coconut Curry with Chickpeas over Jasmine Rice

Day 6
- **Breakfast:** Avocado and Berry Smoothie
- **Lunch:** Spinach and Feta Stuffed Portobello Mushrooms
- **Dinner:** Lemon Garlic Shrimp with Zucchini Noodles

Day 7
- **Breakfast:** Omelette with Spinach, Tomatoes, and Feta
- **Lunch:** Carrot and Coriander Soup
- **Dinner:** Eggplant Moussaka

Week 4

Day 1

- **Breakfast:** Coconut Milk Rice Pudding with Mango
- **Lunch:** Greek Salad with Hummus and Pita Bread
- **Dinner:** Baked Cod with Parsley Pesto and Steamed Carrots

Day 2

- **Breakfast:** Peach and Raspberry Smoothie
- **Lunch:** Cold Beetroot Soup
- **Dinner:** Vegetable Paella

Day 3

- **Breakfast:** Scrambled Tofu with Avocado on Toast
- **Lunch:** Tomato and Cucumber Gazpacho
- **Dinner:** Moroccan Vegetable Tagine with Couscous

Day 4

- **Breakfast:** Chia Seed and Kiwi Pudding
- **Lunch:** Broccoli and Almond Soup
- **Dinner:** Grilled Turkey Burgers with Sweet Potato Fries

Day 5

- **Breakfast:** Apple Cinnamon Oatmeal
- **Lunch:** Zucchini and Yellow Squash Ribbon Salad
- **Dinner:** Stuffed Peppers with Ground Turkey and Quinoa

Day 6

- **Breakfast:** Carrot Orange Smoothie
- **Lunch:** Egg Salad Sandwich on Soft Whole Wheat Bread
- **Dinner:** Spaghetti Squash with Tomato Basil Sauce

Day 7

- **Breakfast:** Cottage Cheese with Fresh Berries
- **Lunch:** Roasted Red Pepper and Tomato Soup
- **Dinner:** Baked Chicken Breast with Mushroom Risotto

Week 5

Day 1

- **Breakfast:** Kiwi and Banana Yogurt Smoothie
- **Lunch:** Avocado Egg Salad on Soft Whole-Grain Bread
- **Dinner:** Lemon Thyme Chicken with Garlic Mashed Potatoes

Day 2
- **Breakfast:** Mixed Berry Compote over Greek Yogurt
- **Lunch:** Sweet Corn and Potato Chowder
- **Dinner:** Quinoa and Black Bean Stuffed Tomatoes

Day 3
- **Breakfast:** Cucumber Melon Smoothie
- **Lunch:** Caprese Salad with Balsamic Reduction
- **Dinner:** Garlic Butter Baked Salmon with Asparagus

Day 4
- **Breakfast:** Baked Avocado Eggs
- **Lunch:** Spinach and Pear Soup
- **Dinner:** Zucchini Lasagna

Day 5
- **Breakfast:** Almond Milk Porridge with Dried Fruit
- **Lunch:** Cucumber, Dill, and Yogurt Salad
- **Dinner:** Cauliflower Steak with Tahini Sauce

Day 6
- **Breakfast:** Mango Lassi Smoothie
- **Lunch:** Curried Lentil Soup
- **Dinner:** Stir-Fried Tofu with Bell Peppers and Broccoli

Day 7
- **Breakfast:** Raspberry and Flaxseed Smoothie
- **Lunch:** Grilled Peach and Chicken Salad
- **Dinner:** Butternut Squash Curry with Basmati Rice

Week 6

Day 1
- **Breakfast:** Pear, Walnut, and Cinnamon Smoothie
- **Lunch:** Chickpea and Avocado Salad
- **Dinner:** Lemon Herb Roasted Chicken with Green Beans

Day 2
- **Breakfast:** Coconut and Pineapple Smoothie
- **Lunch:** Tomato, Basil, and Mozzarella Salad
- **Dinner:** Fish Tacos with Cabbage Slaw

Day 3
- **Breakfast:** Green Tea and Honeydew Smoothie
- **Lunch:** Quinoa Salad with Cucumbers and Mint
- **Dinner:** Vegetarian Shepherd's Pie

Day 4

- **Breakfast:** Blueberry and Almond Butter Smoothie
- **Lunch:** Spiced Pumpkin Soup
- **Dinner:** Stuffed Acorn Squash

Day 5

- **Breakfast:** Strawberry and Cream Cheese Sandwich
- **Lunch:** Kale and Cannellini Bean Soup
- **Dinner:** Parmesan Crusted Chicken with Arugula Salad

Day 6

- **Breakfast:** Banana and Spinach Smoothie
- **Lunch:** Mediterranean Chickpea and Vegetable Wrap
- **Dinner:** Baked Shrimp with Feta and Tomatoes

Day 7

- **Breakfast:** Oatmeal with Pumpkin Puree and Spices
- **Lunch:** Broccoli and Cheese Soup
- **Dinner:** Roasted Vegetable Quiche

Week 7

Day 1

- **Breakfast:** Avocado Kiwi Smoothie
- **Lunch:** Cold Lentil Salad with Cucumbers and Herbs
- **Dinner:** Garlic Lemon Cod with Sauteed Spinach

Day 2

- **Breakfast:** Banana Oatmeal Cups
- **Lunch:** Roasted Cauliflower Soup
- **Dinner:** Honey Mustard Chicken with Roasted Root Vegetables

Day 3

- **Breakfast:** Coconut Yogurt with Honey and Almonds
- **Lunch:** Beet and Orange Salad
- **Dinner:** Vegetable Kebabs with Quinoa Salad

Day 4

- **Breakfast:** Green Apple Smoothie
- **Lunch:** Spicy Sweet Potato Soup
- **Dinner:** Balsamic Glazed Salmon with Steamed Broccolini

Day 5

- **Breakfast:** Ricotta and Honeyed Pear Toast
- **Lunch:** Kale Caesar Salad with Chickpea Croutons
- **Dinner:** Mushroom and Pea Risotto

Day 6

- **Breakfast:** Chilled Berry Soup
- **Lunch:** Caponata on Soft Polenta
- **Dinner:** Grilled Tilapia with Mango Salsa

Day 7

- **Breakfast:** Poached Eggs with Avocado and Spinach on Toast
- **Lunch:** Gazpacho with Melon
- **Dinner:** Ratatouille with Soft Polenta

Week 8

Day 1

- **Breakfast:** Pineapple and Turmeric Smoothie
- **Lunch:** Carrot Slaw with Raisins and Walnuts
- **Dinner:** Lemon Garlic Roasted Chicken with Asparagus

Day 2

- **Breakfast:** Cottage Cheese with Grated Apple and Cinnamon
- **Lunch:** Cucumber and Dill Salad with Smoked Salmon
- **Dinner:** Beef Stew with Soft Cooked Vegetables

Day 3

- **Breakfast:** Toasted Oat and Yogurt Layered Parfait
- **Lunch:** Summer Vegetable Soup
- **Dinner:** Baked Sole with Lemon Caper Sauce and Spinach

Day 4

- **Breakfast:** Papaya and Lime Smoothie
- **Lunch:** Warm Quinoa Salad with Roasted Squash and Pomegranate
- **Dinner:** Chicken Piccata with Soft Noodles

Day 5

- **Breakfast:** Scrambled Eggs with Fresh Herbs on Toast
- **Lunch:** Eggplant and Chickpea Stew
- **Dinner:** Shrimp Scampi over Soft Polenta

Day 6
- **Breakfast:** Pear and Walnut Salad with Yogurt
- **Lunch:** Zesty Quinoa and Bean Salad
- **Dinner:** Stuffed Bell Peppers with Ground Turkey and Vegetables

Day 7
- **Breakfast:** Smoothie with Blueberry, Banana, and Flaxseed
- **Lunch:** Creamy Asparagus Soup
- **Dinner:** Maple Glazed Pork Chops with Apple Slaw

FOOD TRACKER JOURNAL

How do you feel your current diet impacts your Sjogren's Syndrome symptoms? Identify any foods you suspect exacerbate your symptoms.

WATER INTAKE

PERSONAL NOTES

DAYS	BREAKFAST	LUNCH	DINNER
MON			
TUE			
WED			
THU			
FRI			
SAT			
SUN			

FOOD TRACKER JOURNAL

What specific goals do you hope to achieve by following the Sjogren's Syndrome diet? (e.g., reducing dryness, improving energy levels).

WATER INTAKE

PERSONAL NOTES

DAYS	BREAKFAST	LUNCH	DINNER
MON			
TUE			
WED			
THU			
FRI			
SAT			
SUN			

FOOD TRACKER JOURNAL

What challenges do you anticipate facing while adapting to the Sjogren's Syndrome diet, and how do you plan to overcome them?

WATER INTAKE

PERSONAL NOTES

DAYS	BREAKFAST	LUNCH	DINNER
MON			
TUE			
WED			
THU			
FRI			
SAT			
SUN			

FOOD TRACKER JOURNAL

Which nutrients are especially important for managing Sjogren's Syndrome, and why?

WATER INTAKE

PERSONAL NOTES

DAYS	BREAKFAST	LUNCH	DINNER
MON			
TUE			
WED			
THU			
FRI			
SAT			
SUN			

FOOD TRACKER JOURNAL

How do your Sjogren's Syndrome symptoms
change, if at all, when you alter your diet?

WATER INTAKE

PERSONAL NOTES

DAYS	BREAKFAST	LUNCH	DINNER
MON			
TUE			
WED			
THU			
FRI			
SAT			
SUN			

FOOD TRACKER JOURNAL

How do you plan to ensure adequate hydration throughout the day? List some strategies or reminders you could use.

WATER INTAKE

PERSONAL NOTES

DAYS	BREAKFAST	LUNCH	DINNER
MON			
TUE			
WED			
THU			
FRI			
SAT			
SUN			

FOOD TRACKER JOURNAL

Identify any foods you need to eliminate or reduce in your diet. What are some suitable alternatives that you enjoy?

WATER INTAKE

PERSONAL NOTES

DAYS	BREAKFAST	LUNCH	DINNER
MON			
TUE			
WED			
THU			
FRI			
SAT			
SUN			

FOOD TRACKER JOURNAL

How will you manage social situations, dining out, or family meals while sticking to your diet plan?

WATER INTAKE

PERSONAL NOTES

DAYS	BREAKFAST	LUNCH	DINNER
MON			
TUE			
WED			
THU			
FRI			
SAT			
SUN			

FOOD TRACKER JOURNAL

After eating certain foods, have you noticed any changes in how you feel? Identify foods that make you feel better or worse.

....

....

....

....

....

....

....

....

....

WATER INTAKE

PERSONAL NOTES

DAYS	BREAKFAST	LUNCH	DINNER
MON			
TUE			
WED			
THU			
FRI			
SAT			
SUN			

FOOD TRACKER JOURNAL

Changing one's diet can be challenging. How have you adapted to these changes, and what support do you need?

WATER INTAKE

PERSONAL NOTES

DAYS	BREAKFAST	LUNCH	DINNER
MON			
TUE			
WED			
THU			
FRI			
SAT			
SUN			

FOOD TRACKER JOURNAL

Are there any vitamins or supplements recommended for Sjogren's Syndrome that you are considering? What are your thoughts on their potential benefits?

WATER INTAKE

PERSONAL NOTES

DAYS	BREAKFAST	LUNCH	DINNER
MON			
TUE			
WED			
THU			
FRI			
SAT			
SUN			

FOOD TRACKER JOURNAL

Besides diet, what other self-care strategies do you find beneficial for managing your Sjogren's Syndrome?

WATER INTAKE

PERSONAL NOTES

DAYS	BREAKFAST	LUNCH	DINNER
MON			
TUE			
WED			
THU			
FRI			
SAT			
SUN			

FOOD TRACKER JOURNAL

Based on your experience so far, how do you
envision continuing to incorporate the principles
of the Sjogren's Syndrome diet into your lifestyle
long-term?

....
....
....
....
....
....
....
....
....
....

WATER INTAKE

PERSONAL NOTES

____
____
____
____
____
____

DAYS	BREAKFAST	LUNCH	DINNER
MON			
TUE			
WED			
THU			
FRI			
SAT			
SUN			

Scan the QR code below to get a surprise bonus!